Suspension Fitness For Cycling

Suspension Fitness for Cycling

ISBN: 9781797726588

Tracy Christenson: Reno, NV

CONTENTS

Preface

Health-related problems due to obesity, stress, and inactivity are a huge concern for both individuals and society. Furthermore, people are busier than ever. I see the struggles people have trying to balance the immediate demands of everyday life, with a desire to be fit and healthy. Most often, people understand and truly want to be more active, fit, and healthy. However, there is always something competing for time and opportunities, and the immediate need usually takes precedent over a long-term plan for better health and fitness.

I see these struggles in the lives of my friends and clients. I have also experienced these struggles myself through the demands of running a small business, managing advanced education, handling a fixer-upper house full of dogs, and needing to generate income through additional means while building the business (and putting together this book). Even in my case, when I had all the tools and knowledge, it was still tough.

It was tough, but it was doable.

I wanted to bring those tools and knowledge to the people I saw around me who were struggling to bring better health and fitness into their lives. Individuals who truly wanted change but didn't have the resources. Those who didn't have the time available to attend exercise classes or make the trip to the gym several times a week. People who didn't have the resources to hire a personal trainer. People who didn't know where to start.

I also wanted to show people something different. When I go into traditional fitness centers, I still see people walking around through rows of machines, each machine isolating one area of the body. Sometimes they are following a workout routine that they have been doing for months or years. They look bored, they are rarely sweating or breathing even moderately hard, and often they are poorly fitted to the machine. Although training with suspension is not new, I feel it is vastly underused, and most people don't realize the incredible benefits.

When I have introduced a suspension and body-weight training approach to clients or friends, they have been exceptionally receptive.

The following comments really stood out:

> *"This is fun…like water-skiing!"*

> *"The machines at the gym make my wrist hurt, but this feels OK."*

> *"I can really feel this in my core!"*

In addition to working with the general population through personal training, working with a community of cyclists, runners, and triathletes through our cycling studio gave me a whole different perspective. A lot of them actually did have time (although it was often limited) or made time for their training, but it usually wasn't easy. There was also less time left for strength work after their endurance workouts. Because they loved to run or ride, that's what they wanted to do with the time they had, and strength workouts often got pushed off the cliff. Those who did go to the gym often performed programs too reliant on traditional machine work that was less unique to the demands of their endurance activity. Machine work didn't always transfer over in the most efficient way to support their training goals. I wanted to do something for them as well.

Coming Up with a Solution

Training with suspension and your own body weight is a method that works. It's not a gimmick, and it can benefit a wide range of abilities and goals. It's also fun, and it can be done anywhere! I can't think of a better approach for achieving greater strength and fitness, especially for busy professionals, or those looking for better performance, emphasizing moving their body weight, versus moving plates and dumbbells. You achieve more in less time. You improve the ability of your muscles to function together and work as one unit, which transfers most efficiently to real-world physical demands. You can also tailor any workout to your level and goals.

What I love is that this is so useful for so many different fitness populations. Beginners, advanced exercisers, seniors, athletes, stay-at-home moms, working professionals, and post-rehab clients are all people with whom I have used suspension training, and we've experienced successful outcomes. However, until the writing of this book, the information out there was still sparse and inconsistent and not always of the greatest quality. My goal is to display what I use and have been able to share with my clients, to a wider audience, at a lower cost than I could ever offer through group or individual training. I want this book to achieve the following:

Introduce people to a method of achieving better strength and stability to which they have never been exposed.

To make a strength training program more convenient and achievable for those already balancing an endurance training program with all of life's other demands.

Provide motivation to start or continue with resistance training by providing information on the substantial benefits to cycling performance.

Provide direction on a developing strength and stability specific to running. I hope I have been successful in these these areas, and I hope I am able to provide at least some enhancement to your training program.

Introduction

I began my career as a personal trainer at a large fitness center in Dallas, Texas. Early in my time there, I remember seeing one of the more innovative instructors—who was also a cycling and triathlon coach—experiment with a suspension trainer during off-peak hours. This took place in the corner of the fitness center's free-weight area. It was like nothing I had seen before. As a young and relatively new trainer, educated in the traditional approach, combining machines, free weights, and some cardio, I filed this new method away in my mind.

A couple of years later, a little more confident as a strength and conditioning professional and looking to expand my skill set, I purchased my own suspension training kit and started to experiment. A TRX® Suspension Training Certification course came soon after, and I started a gradual but complete shift in my training style for my clients, as well as myself. This change wasn't a conscious move, but the suspension method felt so much better than what I'd been teaching. I gravitated toward it, made it a focus of my fitness program, and it was well received by my clients.

I shifted away from machines and isolation exercises toward a more functional approach to supporting and strengthening whole-body movement patterns we all use in everyday life as well as in our chosen sports. This method requires the body to work as a unit, and I learned ways to develop and improve techniques to achieve this, and then tailor them in unique ways for individuals. Suspension training fits very well into my evolving philosophy of what an outstanding training program should be.

TRX® is the pioneer equipment brand and is the most widely recognized name among many high-quality suspended products available. The equipment is easy to obtain, and with basic setup prices relatively low, suspension training has, not surprisingly, become widely known and practiced across the world in recent years. A significant population of professional and amateur athletes and fitness enthusiasts have heard of it and tried it, and many now even own a suspended trainer. But because it requires a little more technique and body awareness, suspension training has a learning curve and can be a little intimidating to novices.

People with more experience in physical conditioning are often more comfortable self-starting with suspension training, but when those individuals come to me for some fine-tuning or to learn about working very specific movement patterns, I sometimes see fundamental positional errors that have been ingrained through repetition and have become bad habits.

My goal with this book is to provide all the basic information on how to get the most out of this type of training, whether it be as supplemental resistance training for endurance athletes; as a means of achieving general fitness to assist with overall well-being and daily life; or a short, do-anywhere workout for business travelers for whom something is a lot better than nothing. Resources in this book will guide you in learning to use suspension training in the gym, at home, or on the road.

I hope this book helps you discover the rewards of suspension training and that you achieve the same success with it as my clients and I have.

How to Use This Book

Section 1: Chapters 1–4

This section covers essential information about the basics of using a suspended strainer. The general concepts covered include equipment setup, the progression in adjusting resistance and stability levels, technique, external loading, and how to be comfortable training with suspension anywhere, at any level, and for any objective.

Section 2: Chapter 5-6

This section contains specific information on how strength training benefits cycling and on developing a cycling specific strength program.

Section 3: Exercise Libraries

This section contains a libary of strength movements, as well as some foundation and cycling specific workouts that can be done using your suspended trainer.

Section 1

Setup and Technique

Chapter 1

Origins and Development

Using suspension using your own body weight to improve flexibilty and mobility is the primary focus of this book. Suspension training can also be used to improve strength, balance, and endurance and sports performance, and more information can be found on these benefits in the Complete Suspension Fitness book.

Training with suspension is not new, but it has evolved and is being more widely recognized as a valuable and useful tool. Evidence of rope training dates back to the mid-1800s for many athletes, while gymnasts and trapeze artists have long performed aspects of their sports using suspension. If you have ever watched the "rings" competition in gymnastics, you have seen a form of suspension training.

Since the mid-1990s, a variety of suspended training systems have been commercially available to professional trainers, home users, and the like. The most popular and widely recognized system is the TRX® Suspension Trainer.

The suspension exercises and concepts discussed in this book are not limited to the TRX® Suspension Trainer, but can be practiced with a variety of suspension training brands available at a range of price points. Training with suspension is a great strength training tool, but can also be used in a variety of ways to improve flexibility and mobility. Although the setup for both uses is the same, this book will focus on primarily on flexbility training.

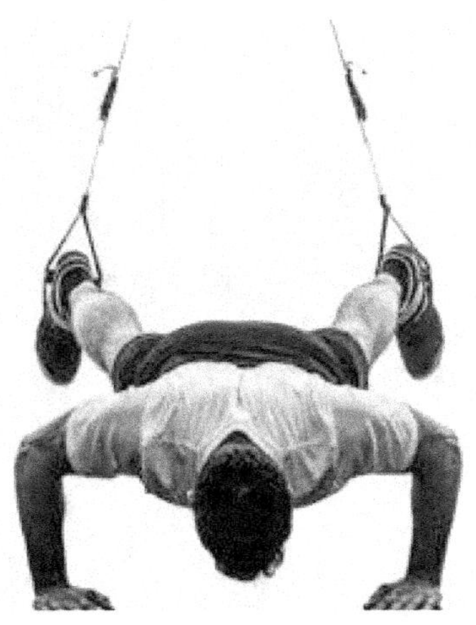

What it is

Suspension training uses your own body weight through the movements and stretches you will learn about in this book. It is portable, extremely versatile, and can be used for building and flexibility and mobility anywhere. You can also focus on specific areas of the body, or perform exercises that develop mobilty throughout the whole body by combining movements together. Most movements in suspension training can be easily modified to suit a variety of fitness and ability levels.

Novice exercisers will appreciate the joint-friendly and easily adjustable resistances offered by the movements. Those at advanced fitness levels will appreciate the progressions and easy transitions between movements. Those using suspension training notice significant gains in the performance of everyday activities, strength and stabilty, and even through athletic endevers. When your quality of movement improves, you feel better, move better and can perform better.

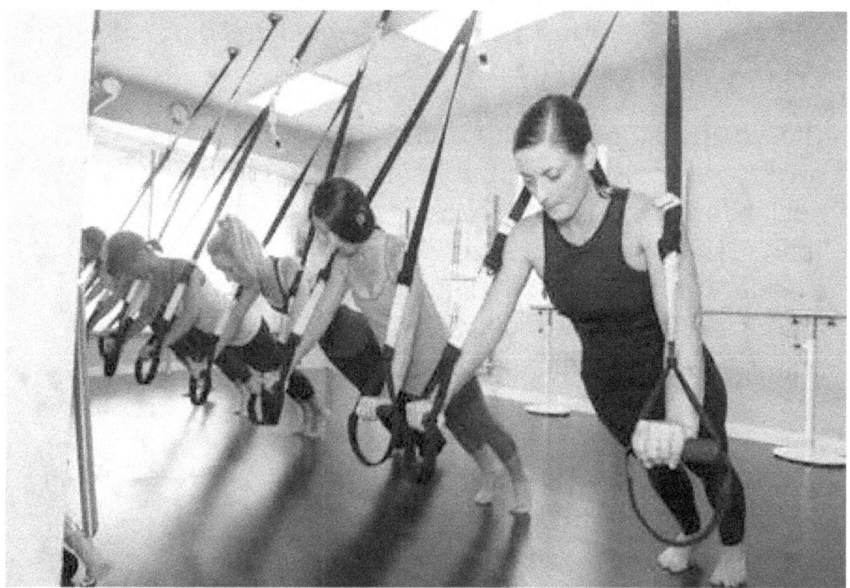

Suspended Training Is Appropriate for All Ability Levels

Suspended training makes body-weight training accessible to a broad spectrum of abilities. This is because the resistance levels are so easy to adjust. When you are hanging on the straps, whatever percent of your body weight is being supported by the straps is the weight with which you will ultimately be working. This could range from a small percent, resulting in a very light load, or the weight of your entire body. Your body position relative to the straps and the ground will determine how much weight with which you will be working. I will talk more about that in the upcoming chapters. You can also adjust on the fly if you didn't get the most appropriate resistance at the start of the set or want to work with increasing or decreasing amounts of resistance during your set. Although many of the concepts do apply to strength training, they can also be used in stretching movements. In many of the movements you are able to adjust the level of the stretch by increasing or decreasing the amount of body weight suspensed, as well as changing the angles of the body in relation to the suspension trainer. This makes it a versatile tool for people at many different ability and mobility levels.

Suspended Training Is Ergonomic

Performance coach Mike Gillette talked about the ergonomics of suspension training in his book *Rings of Power*, and he described how this aspect had benefited him.[4] As his age advanced, he began to experience painful shoulder, elbow, and wrist problems in his training. After transitioning to suspension training through rings, he was gradually able to perform pain-free workouts. Training with rings, he wrote, reshaped his approach to strength training and allowed him to once again train hard without pain.

A suspended trainer works in a very comparable manner to the rings with which Mike Gillette had such success. It appears to be joint friendly, because it does not lock you into any set position as you move. The ability to constantly adjust your position during the movement, allows for the optimal amount of flexibility, and freedom of movement. When using a bar or machine, you are usually locked into a fixed position throughout that movement. This includes many of the stretching machines you will find on the market today as well. This focused positioning can overly stress joints as you pass through the range of motion. A suspended system provides the freedom to rotate your wrist and hands around more as needed. This results in less stress transferred through the joints, and often less pain for those with joint discomfort.

A Note for Those Suffering Joint Pain

Mike Gillette's book is a compelling anecdotal account. If you experience joint pain, there are no guarantees a suspended trainer will eliminate discomfort. But I do believe that it will increase the chances of being able to perform movements with less pain. In addition, several of my own clients, who struggle with joint pain, can successfully perform movements on a suspended trainer, that they are unable to perform without pain using other variations, machines, or tools.

> *A suspended trainer gives the hands, wrists, and arms greater scope to rotate and adjust as needed throughout the movement.*

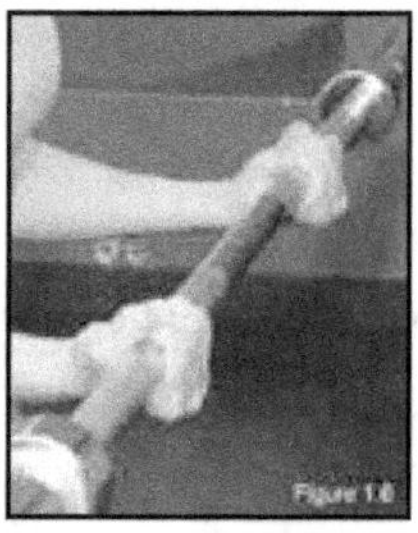

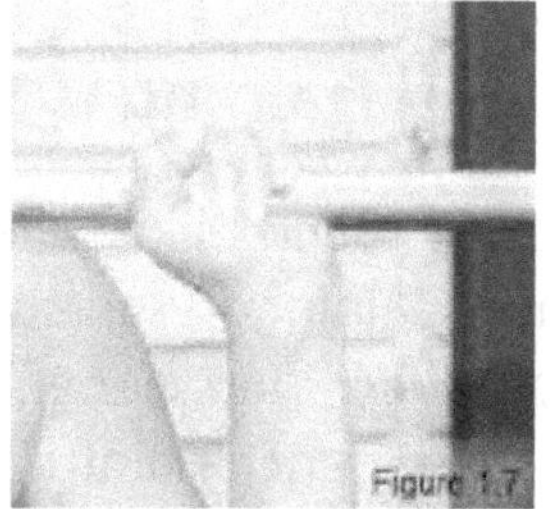

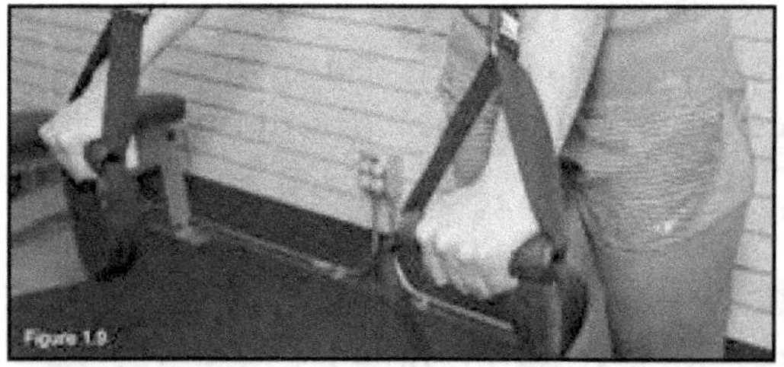

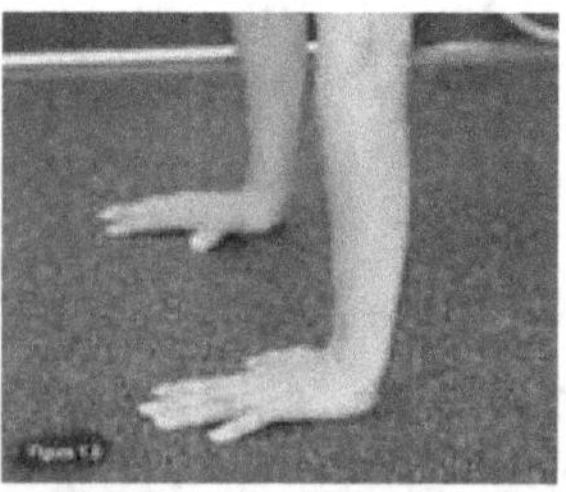

Suspended Training Is Functional

The strength gained from suspension training helps in everyday activities, as well as your chosen sport. The key is that almost every movement in suspension training requires the use of core muscles to stabilize or move the body. In addition, it works the body as a unit. Too often, when you go into a fitness center, you'll see a line of machines… all designed to exercise or stretch distinct parts of the body. For example, you may go through a bicep curl, triceps contraction, chest press, and leg extension as part of your circuit. For most of these, you might be seated with a backrest so you can focus on just the targeted muscle.

This is not how the body moves during everyday tasks, and it's not how I would recommend training. You are missing out on the development of critical motor patterns that go along with the acquired strength. In addition, you are not learning stability or how to use your core to create a solid center of mass that your extremities can rely on, to both transfer force and hold proper alignment when required to lift or move objects. This is especially true when handling asymmetrical loads (such as picking up a heavy bag of groceries, a suitcase, or a small, wiggling dog). It doesn't matter how many plates you can chest press, if you throw out your back when moving a piece of furniture or picking up your child. You may suffer injury if your core doesn't know how to properly activate and stabilize the load you're trying to support with your arms and shoulders. Training your body in suspension will better prepare you to handle the demands of your chosen current fitness endeavors, and the physical demands of everyday living activities.

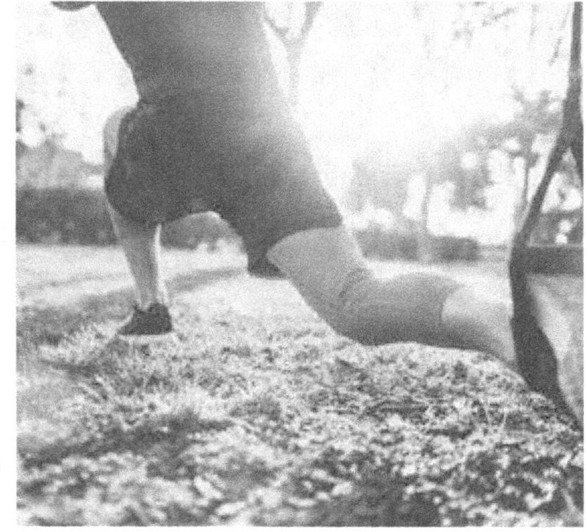

Suspended Training Is Time Effective

There's no traveling between machines with suspended training. It's all right in front of you. Those who are pressed for time will appreciate the quick transition from one movement to the next without lag time.

This time efficiency gives you a lot of bang for your buck. This is especially true if your objective is to perform a dynamic stretch routine that elevates your heart rate, burns more calories per unit of time, and replaces some of the more traditional cardio activities. In addition, it can be much more dynamic and fun. Because the equipment is lightweight and packs up easily, you can also take it with you on the road when traveling, use is outdoors on nice weather days, or supplement your run or crosstraining activity

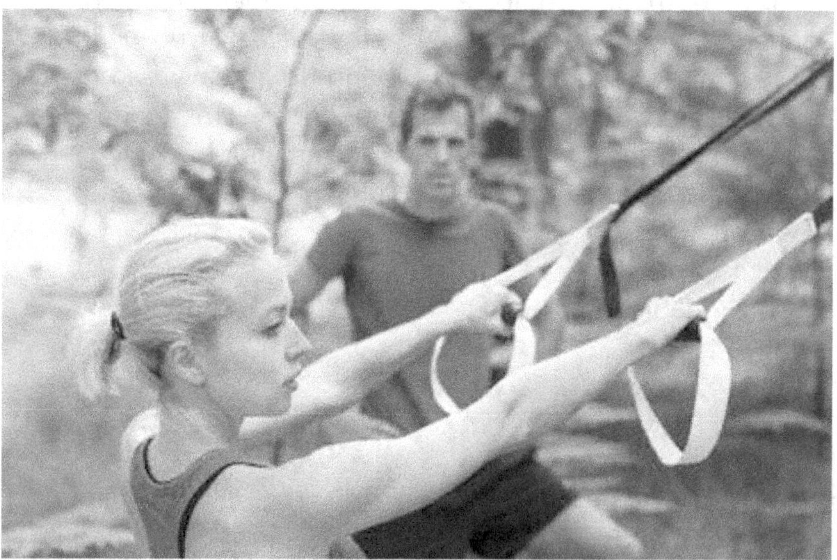

Chapter 2

Getting Set Up and Getting Started

Suspended trainer users can set up their equipment in a variety of ways, both indoors and out. In this chapter I talk a little about each venue and give you some examples. I'm using a TRX Suspension Trainer as an example. If you're using another brand, there may be some slight differences in the features, but the general principles should be the same.

Home Setup

The simplest way to set up a suspended trainer inside your home is to use a door anchor. Some trainers will come with one, but if not, they are readily available online. If you're buying a door anchor separately, or even making your own, make sure it's solid enough to sufficiently support your body weight. I say this because some door anchors are made for anchoring bands, and I would not recommend using one of those for a suspended trainer. A standard door anchor will have a hard, square-shaped block attached to a nylon loop, as in figure 2.1.

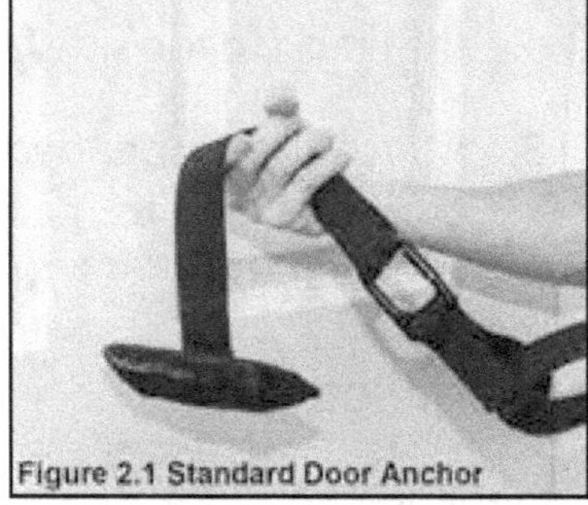

Figure 2.1 Standard Door Anchor

Some people opt for more permanent anchoring solutions (figure 2.2), which bolt onto a wall or beam and are available ready-made as kits. Others prefer to fashion their own using an I-bolt from the local hardware store. If making your own, be sure it's long enough to be inserted to a depth sufficient to hold

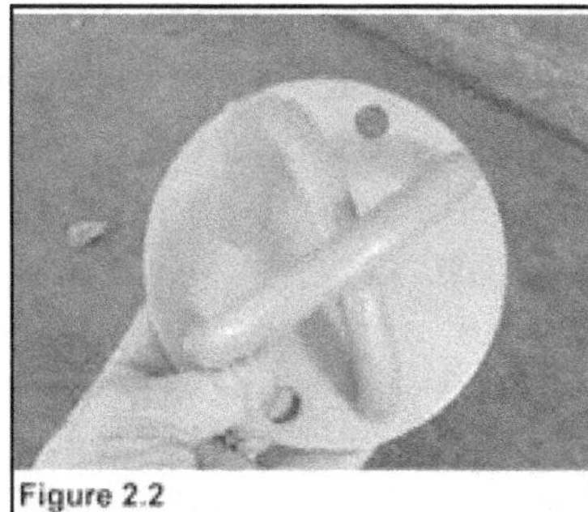

Figure 2.2
Suspension Training Mount

Door Anchor Setups

I strongly advise you to set up your workout space with the door closing toward you. This gives a much stronger support for your equipment and prevents the scenario of the door not being completely secured and possibly opening toward you when you're working out on the suspended trainer.

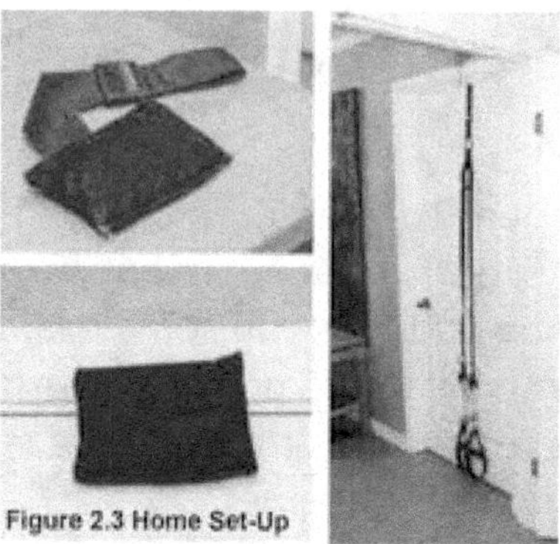
Figure 2.3 Home Set-Up

1. Choose a suitable door with enough space for your workout. You will need a good eight to ten feet of clear space in front   the door.

2. Place the hard square on the back side of the door, midway along the top edge, with the nylon strap feeding through the crack, to the side facing you (figure 2.3). Close the door.

3. Attach the suspended trainer to the nylon loop. Tug on it once or twice to make sure it's secure before beginning your workout!

Outdoor Setups

Outdoor venues offer a variety of options. Trees, fences, poles, beams, and playground equipment can provide good anchoring points for your equipment (figures 2.4 and 2.5). Just make sure whatever you fasten it to won't flex, is securely bolted down, and is strong enough to support the load you'll place on it. Always err on the side of caution. There are times you may need an

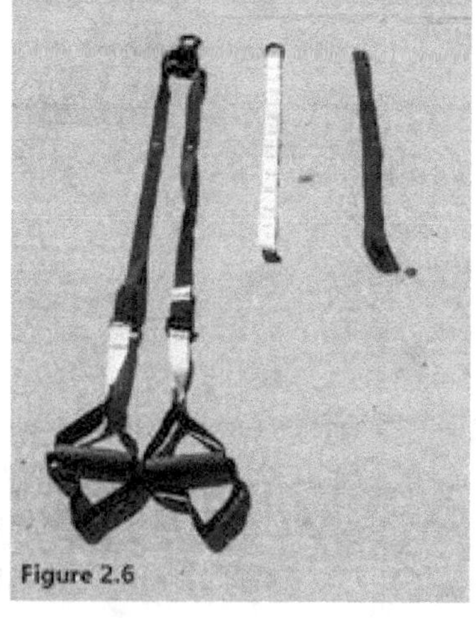
Figure 2.6

extender if you are anchoring high up, or if you need to wrap around something thick such as a beam or thick pole (figure 2.5). Special extender straps for suspended trainers are commercially available, but webbing made for rock climbers works equally well and will provide multiple small loops to clip onto. Figure 2.6 shows three pieces included as part of one training kit: the straps, the anchoring extender, and an extra extender like what is used in

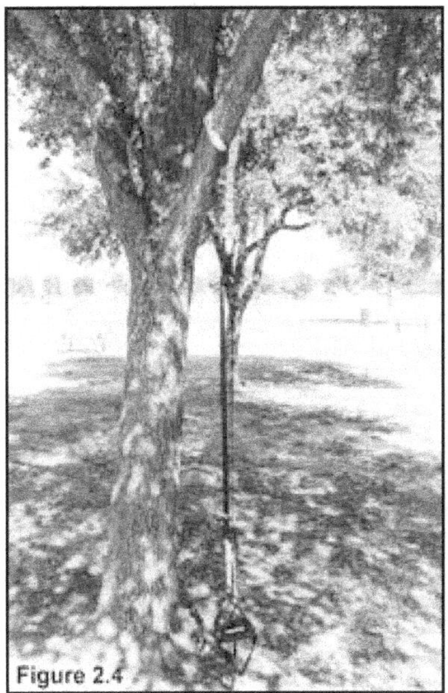

Figure 2.4

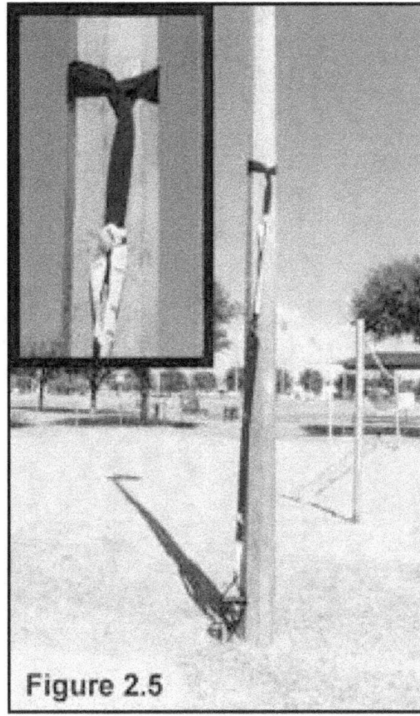

Figure 2.5

figure 2.5. If possible, try to set up your suspended training equipment, so the handles hang about six inches off the ground when the straps are fully extended. If that's not possible, just try and get it as close to six inches as you can.

Lengthening and Shortening Your Suspended Trainer

Most suspended trainers will have a buckle enabling you to adjust the strap length. For the purpose of my examples, I'm using the TRX brand, so if you are using a different brand, just be aware there may be some slight differences in the type of buckles used.

Shorten the strap by pushing the buckle down and pulling the yellow adjustment tab up to the desired height (figures 2.7 and 2.8).

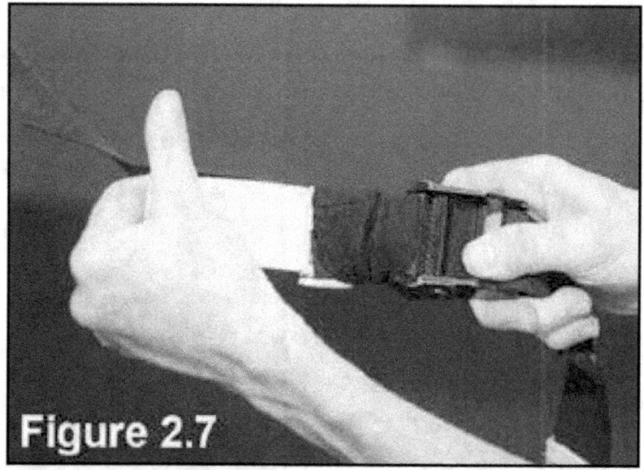

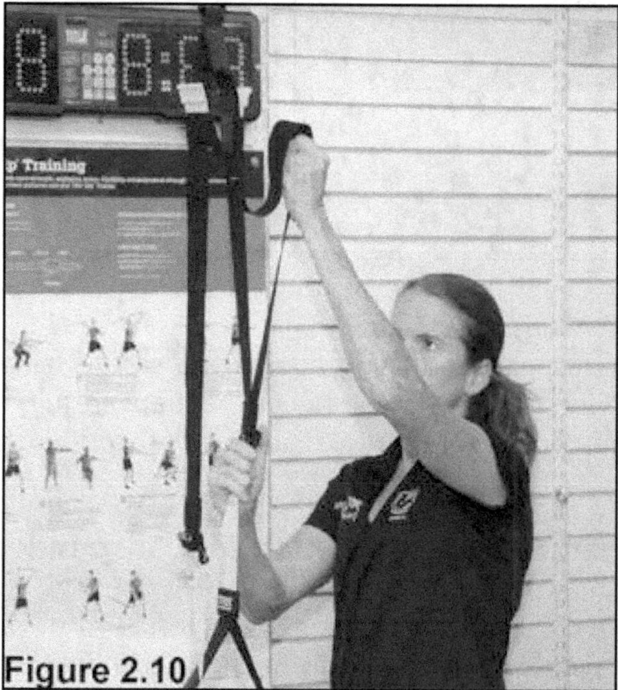

Figure 2.10. To adjust to the super-short length, pull up on the outside strap and then allow it to remain loose, hanging down on the sides like dog ears.

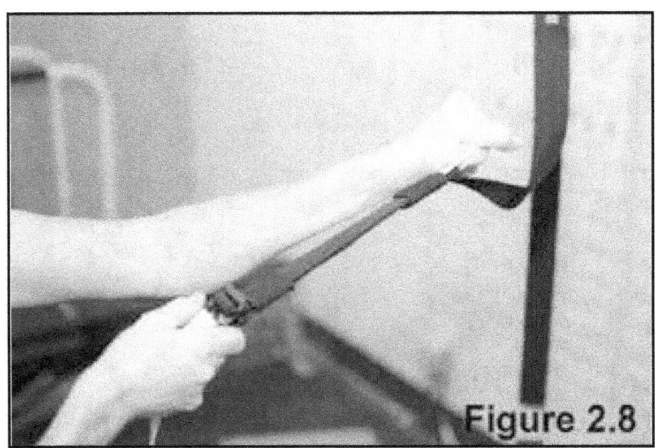

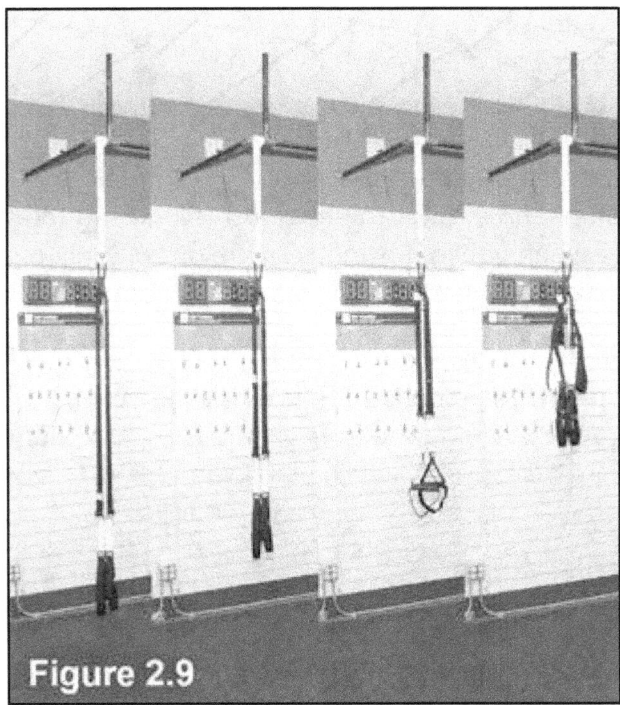

Figure 2.9. Four primary strap lengths: fully extended, mid-length, short, and super-short.

Using a Single Handle Only

Some movements require, or may work best if you to use only one of the handles.

Depending on your suspended training equipment, you might need to tie the handles together to create a single handle. One way to find out is by checking the top of your suspended trainer. If you have a nylon loop at the very top that prevents you from pulling one strap down more than a couple of inches past the other, you probably won't have to adapt your straps to single-handle mode. However, if your equipment doesn't have this loop, you will pull one side all the way through if you pull on just the single opposite handle. You can prevent this by using the single-handle mode when you're putting your weight on only one side. Either way, make sure and test the load before doing the exercise.

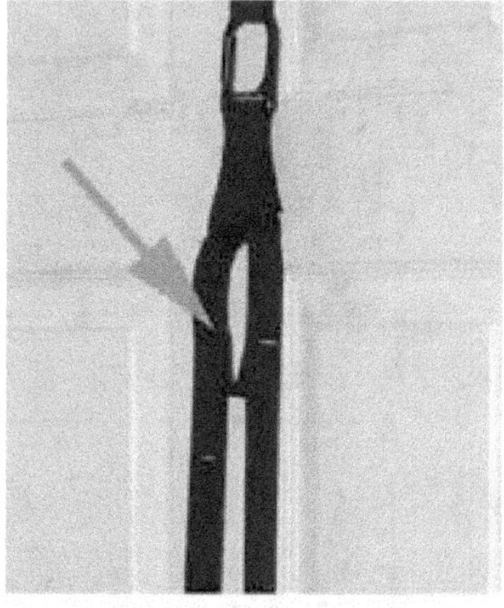

Figure 2.12 Anchoring loop

Currently, all of my own suspended trainers have anchoring loops. I still prefer to use single-handle mode, however, because it keeps the strap not being used from swinging around during the movement I am performing, which can be annoying.

Single-Handle Mode

To tie the handles together:

1. Hold one handle in each hand. The one in your right hand is handle one; the one in your left hand is handle two.

2. Put handle one through the triangle of handle two, and then switch hands. Handle two is now in your right hand (figure 2.11).

3. Repeat this action by putting handle two through handle one.

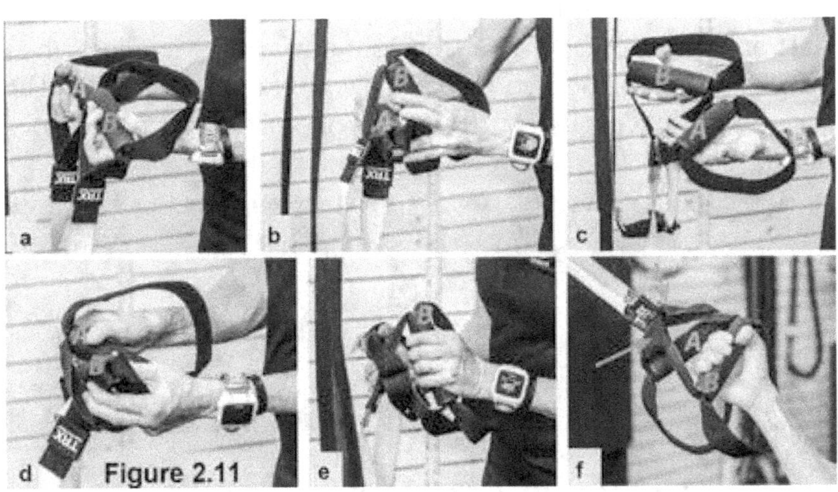

Figure 2.11

Safety Note

If you are working with a suspended trainer without an anchoring loop, it's critical that you hold the correct handle when in single-handle mode. The webbing attached to the handles should look like a mustache, right above the handle you are holding (figure 2.11). Grabbing the incorrect handle could result in one handle slipping through the other during the exercises, which would cause the tie to come undone, possibly resulting in a fall during the movement. Models of suspended trainers with an anchoring loop at the top avoid this, by preventing the straps from being pulled all the way down on one side (figure 2.12).

Using the Foot Cradles

Foot cradles enable you to perform many of the movements in the lying position, either face down or up. For movements where you start on your back, you will place your heels in the cradles. When lying on your stomach, you will place your toes in the cradles. The easiest way I have found to get in each of those positions is shown below.

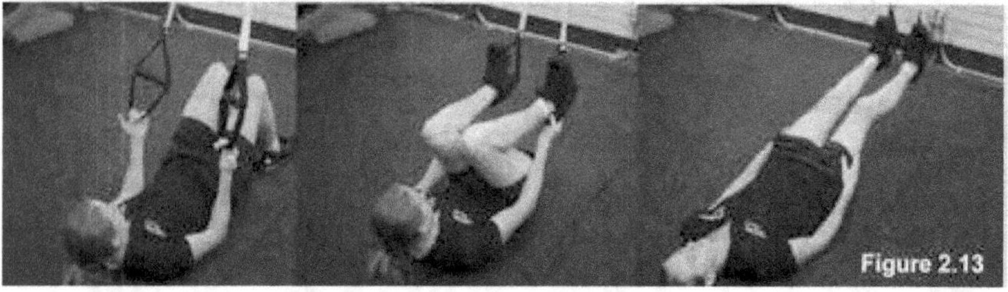

Figure 2.13 Putting your heels in the cradles

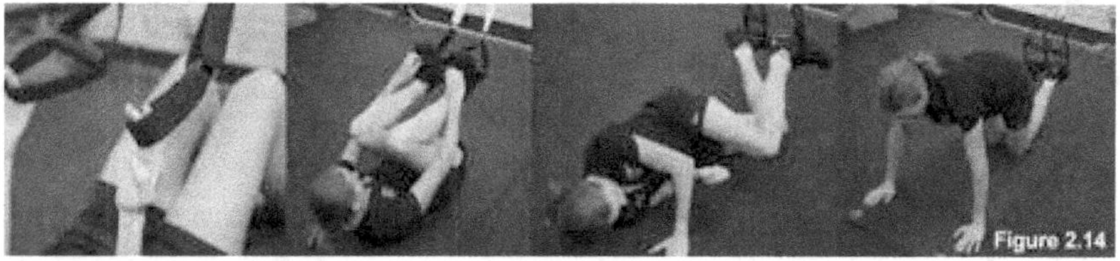

Figure 2.14 Putting your toes in the cradles

Conclusion

In this chapter, I covered the basics of setting up your suspended training equipment, the single-handle mode, and use of the foot cradles. These are the basics of your equipment setup and should give you the tools to be able to set up your trainer anywhere. You can adjust the length, and make use of the foot cradles for floor-based movements. With this information, you will be able to

Chapter 3

Adjusting Resistance Levels

In this chapter, you will learn how to use your body position to modify exercises that match your fitness level and challenge you appropriately. Much of this applies to the strength training movements. However, the concepts of using body positioning to adjust both the resistance and stability levels on a suspended trainer are basic fundamentals and important to achieving proper technique, no matter what the objective of the movement is. In this chapter, we go over how to do this by increasing and decreasing both the resistance and the stability of the movements you perform standing up. Finally, I will talk about how to modify the difficulty level of movements you perform from the ground position

Changing the Resistance Level from the Standing Position

Most movements will have you starting in a standing position. From this position, you can use the angles of your body position to load varying percentages of your body weight onto the straps. This allows a beginner to safely and easily make adjustments to find his or her starting point. It also allows a more experienced user to increase the resistance, as well as perform sets of varying resistance, without interruption. Finally, it allows several users of various abilities to do the same workout together, yet perform the movements at their individual levels of resistance. I find this pretty cool! There is no need to take off or put on weight plates, mess with machines, or trade in dumbbells. You can make these changes quickly and even mid-set if needed.

On the following pages are two examples of how you can change the resistance. One example is of a pushing movement. The other example is of a pulling movement.

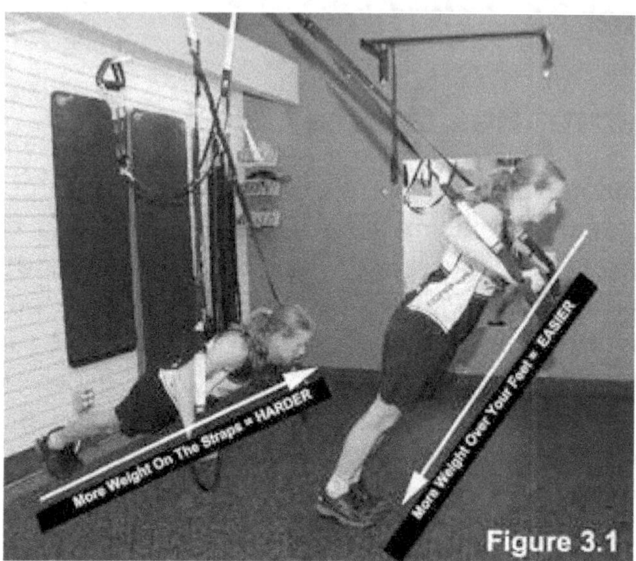

Figure 3.1. Above is an example of two levels of resistance during a suspended push-up. The more upright you are, the more body weight you're supporting with your legs and not having to push with your arms. If you want more resistance, simply step back farther to load more weight onto the straps. All the angles between the hardest (most horizontal) and the easiest (most upright) can

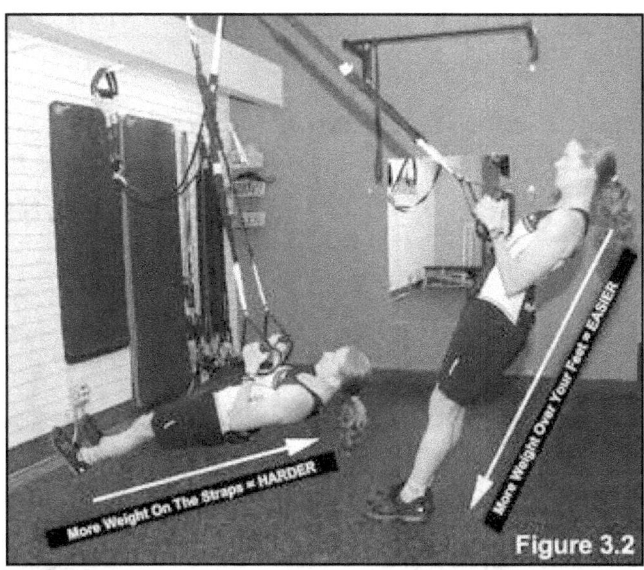

Figure 3.2. Above demonstrates the same concepts during a rowing (pulling) exercise. The farther you step underneath the straps, the more weight is hanging on the straps that you will have to pull up during the movement.

Changing the Resistance Level from the Ground Position

You can adjust the resistance to some degree, from the ground-based position, by changing where you are in relation to the point directly underneath the anchor.

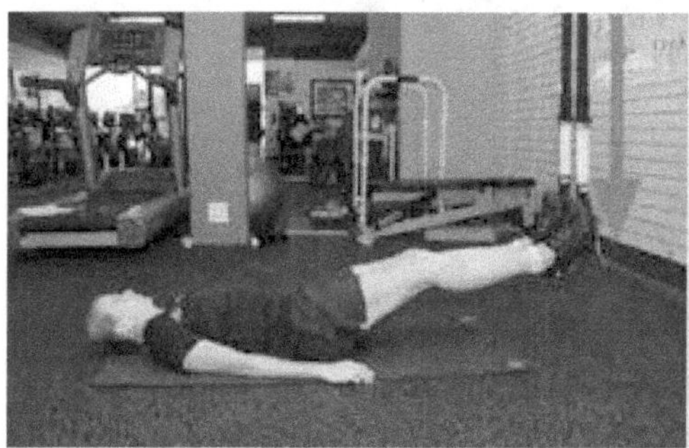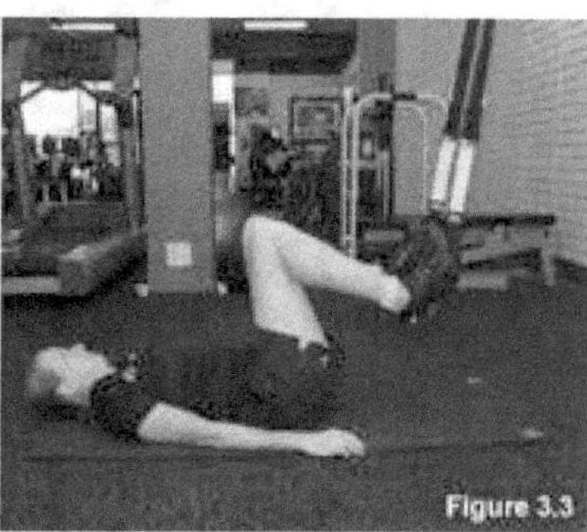

When you're doing movements with your feet in the cradles, you can use your position relative to the center spot, right under the anchor and gravity, to add or reduce resistance.

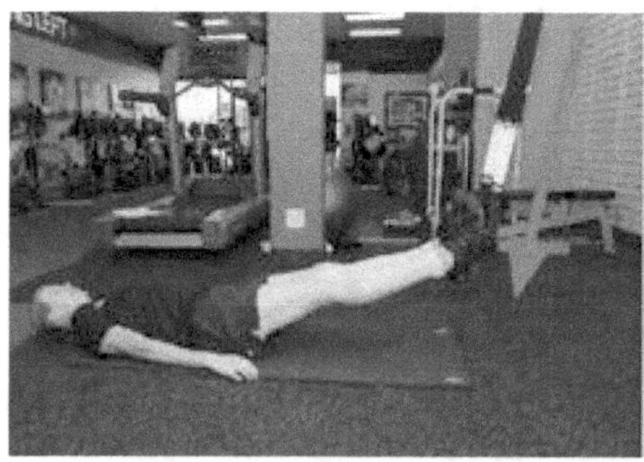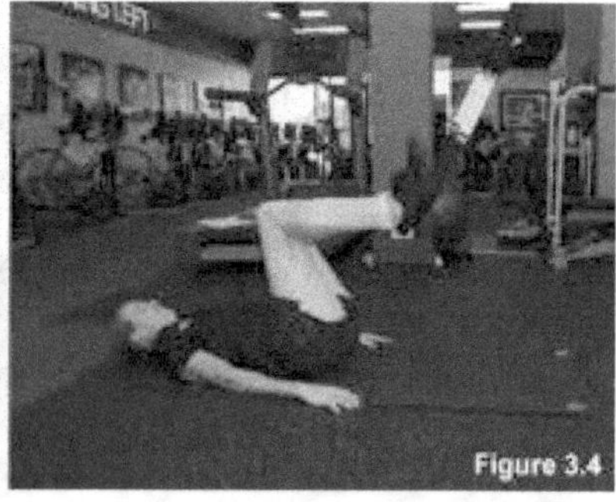

Moving out, so that your starting position is in front of the anchor point, will start the movement at a higher level of resistance. You will be pulling against gravity during the movement, making it harder (see figure 3.4).

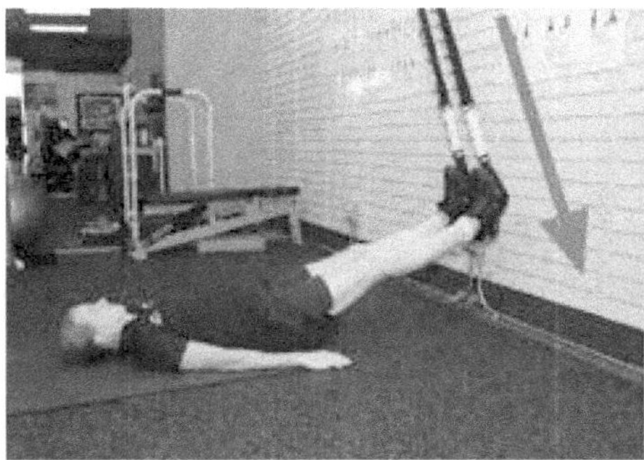 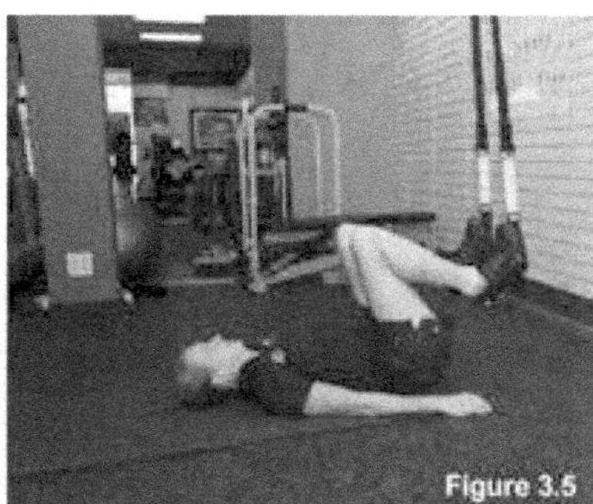

Moving further underneath the anchor point will have the opposite effect. You will be pulling with gravity until the point where you cross neutral (see figure 3.5).

Adjusting the Level of Stability

The instability of suspended training is much of what makes it so highly functional and relevant, to both everyday movements, and to the movement demands of cyclists and runners. Stability can be added or taken away, depending on where your feet are during your standing position. If you are a novice at suspension training, start with the most stable foot position until you feel comfortable with the movement.

The following pages show three examples of how you can adjust the level of stablity by where you place you feet.

- **Wide base of support** *Figure 3.6*: Stability is maximized with a broad base of support and your center of gravity in the middle of that base. If you are performing a push-up and have a wide stance, you will be more stable during that exercise, and it will be easier to balance than if you have a narrow stance.

- **Narrow your support base when using a suspended trainer** *Figure 3.7*: If you would like to challenge your ability to stabilize yourself, bring your feet closer together to create a narrow stance, or do the exercise on just one foot. Decreasing the distance between your feet, decreases the width of the base upon which you are standing. This will be more challenging to your stability, because you are performing the movement on a narrower base of support.

- **Offset stance** *Figure 3.8:* Place one foot in front of the other. An offset stance gives you more stability going from front to back and allows you to shift weight forward and back during the movement. It's a convenient way to self-spot when performing movements with tougher angles. A longer offset position will provide more stability than a shorter one. As with the narrow and wide foot positions shown in figure 3.8, you can adjust your foot placement as needed before or during the movement.

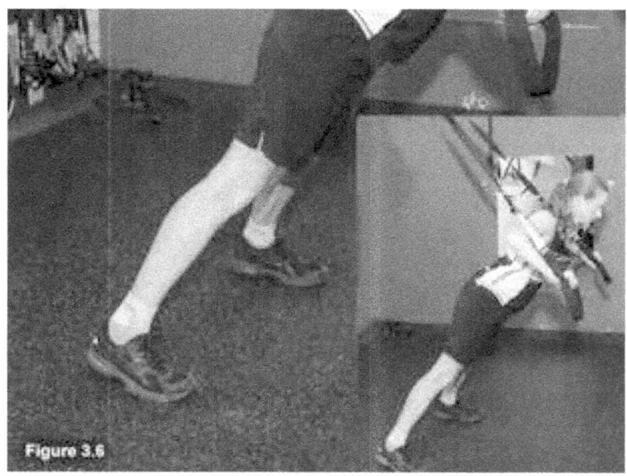

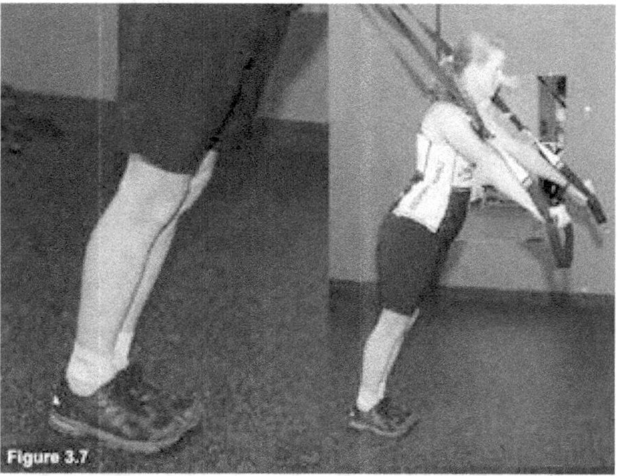

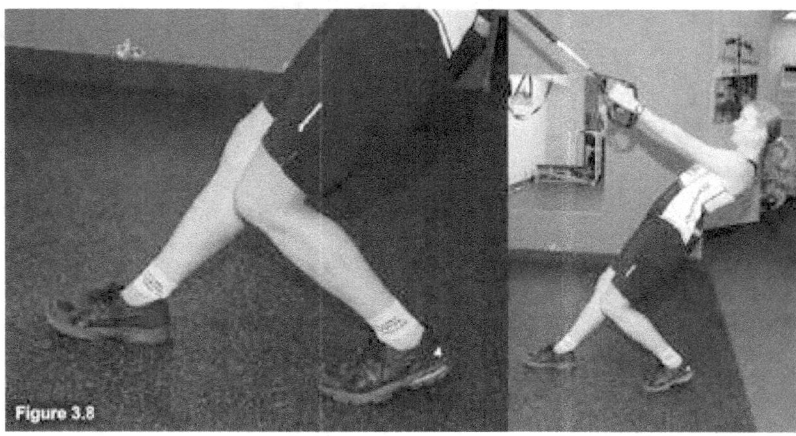

If you are using suspension training for the first time: It's OK to be conservative until you feel comfortable with it. If you're doing an exercise for the first time, start with a position in which you can do about 15 repetitions. It's OK to adjust your position as many times as you need until you feel you're fatiguing your muscles within your goal repetition range while still being able to execute the movement with good form.

If you have a specific workout goal: Choose a resistance level that fits your goal. If you're training for strength, go with a high amount of resistance. If you are looking for more of a cardio, calorie-burning workout, get in a position that loads a lower amount of resistance on your suspended trainer so you can perform the exercise for longer or perform several exercises consecutively.

Now that you know how to make quick ajustments on your suspended trainer, account for this during your workout. For example, if you wanted to add some stretches in between sets of a strenth workout, you can quickly adjust the straps, angles or positions to account for any movement you choose into include in your workout.

> *Tip: To increase the intensity within one movement, perform a drop set. Start with a resistance where you can only do 4 to 5 reps with good form. At that point, adjust your position to make it just easier enough to do another 4 to 5 reps. Adjust your position again, and finish with one last block of 5 reps. Ouch. Your muscles will thank you later.*

Chapter 4

Proper Technique

Perfecting Your Form

The term "form" in suspended training is so important that it's worth defining. "Form" is the exact shape and position of the entire body, from head to toe, and includes specific parts of the body when performing suspended training moves.

Having correct form during suspended training movements is extremely important. To help demonstrate some fundamentals of correct form, I will use a traditional isometric (static) exercise popularly called the "plank." Many people have heard of the "plank" and have experience using it in a training program.

How to Properly Perform a Plank:

1. Start in a ground position facing down.

2. Consciously contract all the muscles you can feel, from your toes to your shoulders.

3. Raise your body up as one unit, so you are contacting the ground with only your forearms and toes.

4. Make sure your body forms a straight line from your shoulders to your ankles.

5. Engage your core by sucking your belly button into your

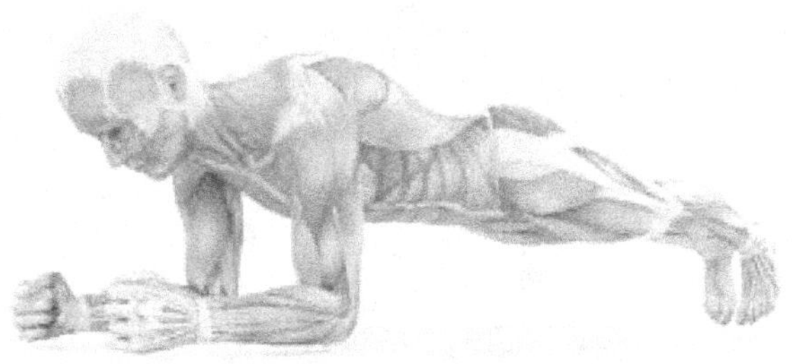

If you have never done the plank, practice it several times over three to four workout sessions before starting a suspended training program. Suspended training requires that you have a good feeling for engaging the core muscles as demanded by correct performance of the plank. If you have done the plank in the past but not recently, a little refresher would be good to reinforce the muscle memory. Time yourself, and focus on increasing the number of seconds you can hold this position. You should aim for at least thirty to sixty seconds before progressing to a more advanced variation such as the suspended plank.

Just Starting Out?

If you are new to strength training, or if it has been a while since you've done it, go ahead and start with a modified version of the plank until your body develops the strength and ability to hold the harder version. To do the modified version, simply hold the position from your knees instead of your toes as shown in figure 4.1. When you can properly hold this position for a full minute, progress to your toes. Initially, reduce the amount of time you attempt to hold the plank when you move up to the more challenging position. Make it a goal to increase your time by five seconds each week until you reach one minute. At this point, you may move to the suspended trainer. Don't rush the progressions, and give your body time to increase its strength and stability during each one.

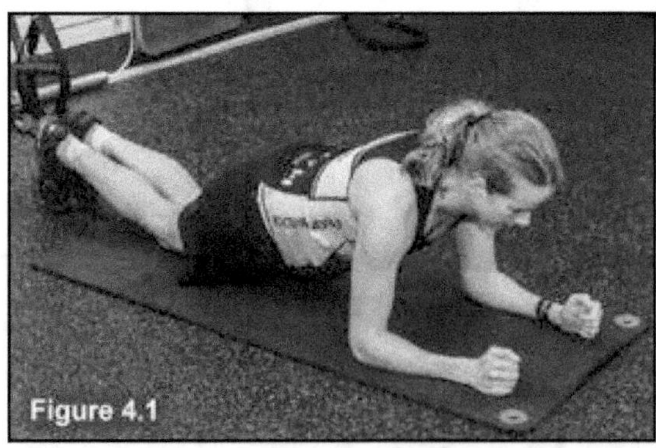

Figure 4.1

Why Does the Plank Matter If We Are Doing Suspension Training?

Performing a plank correctly, gives your body the foundation of muscle control needed for most movements that you will perform on a suspended trainer. You need to stabilize your core, while your arms and legs have the job of moving the weight of your body. Your body will need to know how to properly engage the right muscles in the correct order, and have the strength to hold the position throughout the movement. Losing your plank during a movement on the suspended trainer will result in losing your form.

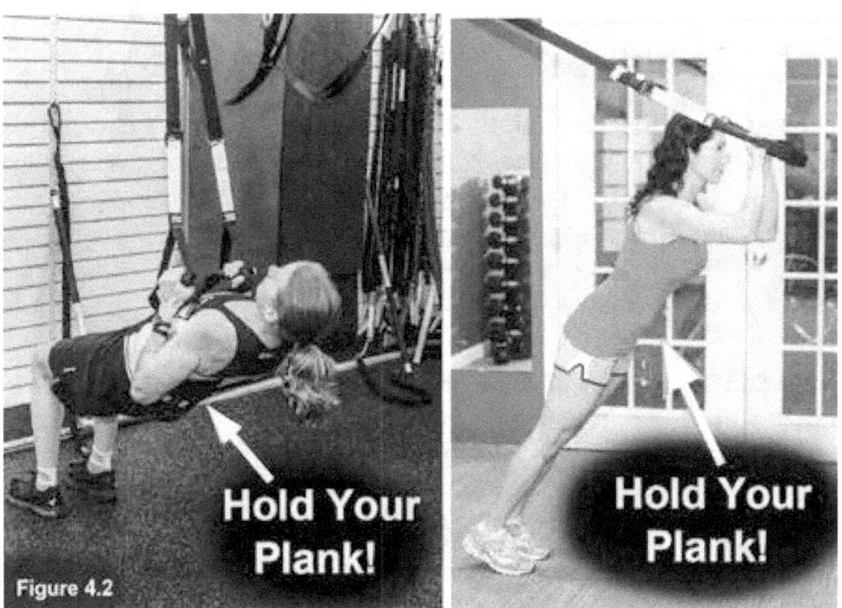

Suspended Training Technique and Common Form Errors

Many beginners make the same mistakes at first with their technique. I will point these errors out here, so you'll know not to make them! Incorrect starting position is often where problems begin, so get this right, and you'll be on a good track. Lack of

Hips: Both poor form and good form of the hips are shown above in figure 4.3. Keep a straight body, like a board. Avoid sagging or having slack in the midsection. Avoid allowing your hips to be up in the air.

Shoulders: Avoid shrugging during the movement, like in figure 4.4. Keep the shoulders down. To help with this, think about maintaining space between your ears and shoulders, and pulling your shoulder blades down toward your butt. Also, lift your chest and maintain good posture in a stand-up-straight type of way.

Core: Keep a tight core, beginning before you even start the movement, until you are finished. Contract and preload the muscles in your abdomen as if someone is going to punch you in the stomach. Pulling your belly button to your spine is also an analogy I use with people. Also, envision making your body as straight as a surfboard or table.

Head and Neck: Keep alignment of the head with the spine. A common error is to look down or up, which often causes other poor posture habits, such as a rounded back and shoulders. See figure 4.5 for examples of poor form and good form of the head and neck.

Wrists: Keep your wrists straight. Avoid a soft wrist, where you allow your wrist to bend back during the movement. See figure 4.6 for examples of poor wrist form and good wrist form.

Knees: For the most part, your knees will maintain alignment with your hips and feet. They should not cave inward or bow outward during squatting or lunging movements, and they should stay centered over your feet during most of those movements. Figure 4.7 shows a common error of form, allowing the hips to drop back on a split-squat movement, resulting in the knee being misaligned with the foot.

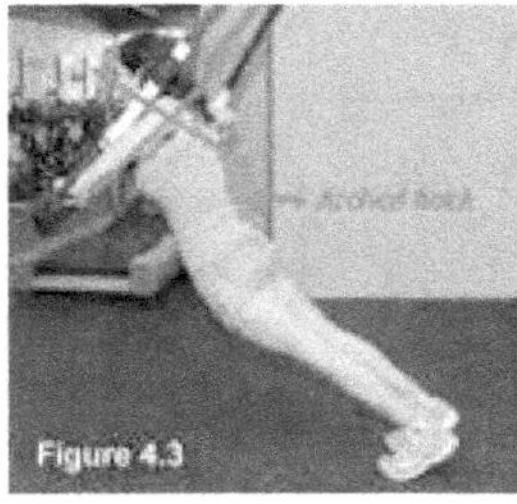
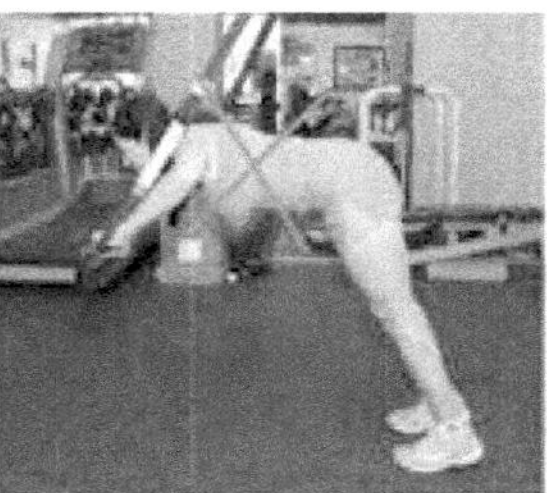
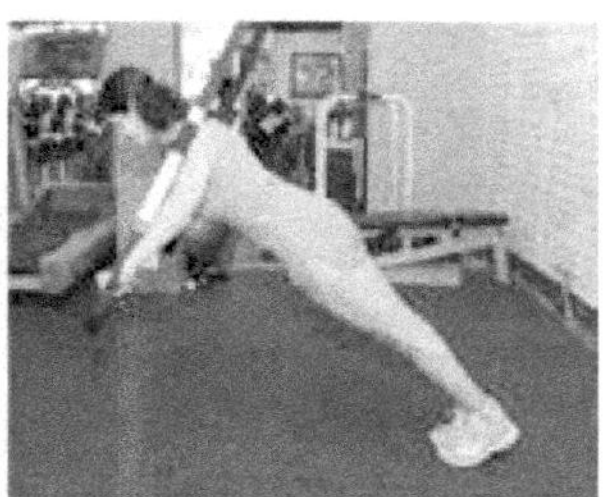

Figure 4.3

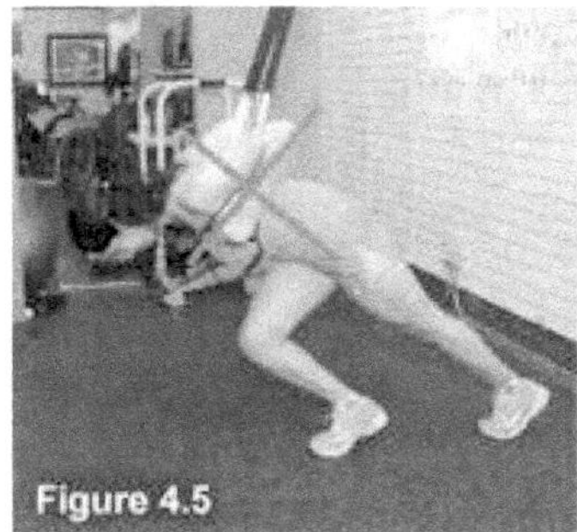
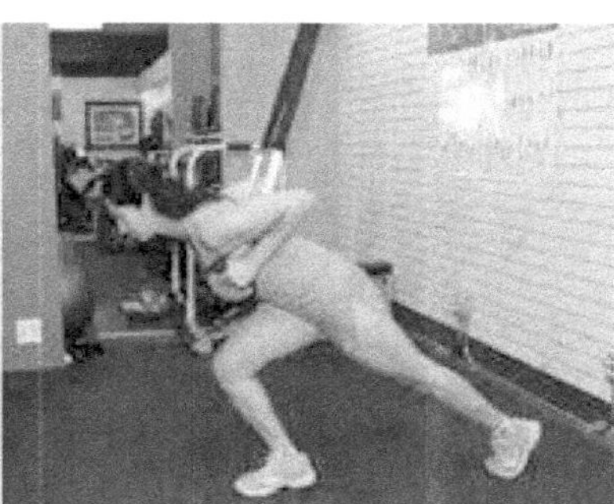

Figure 4.5

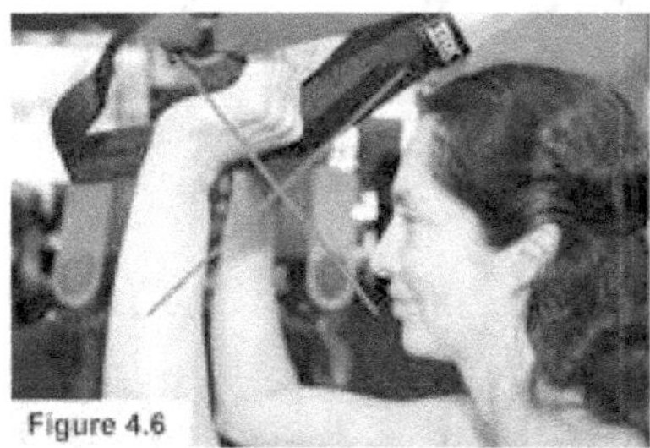
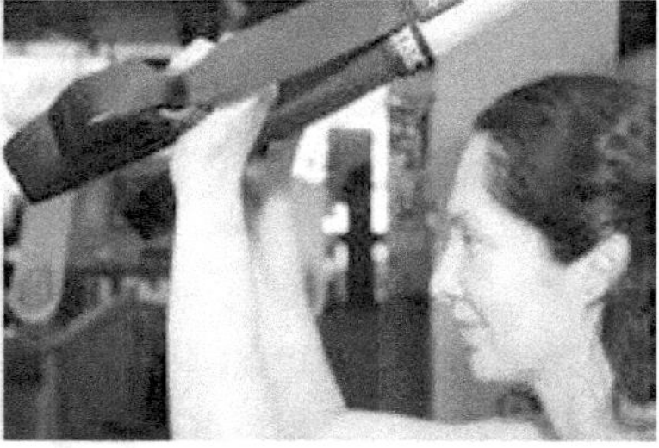

Figure 4.6

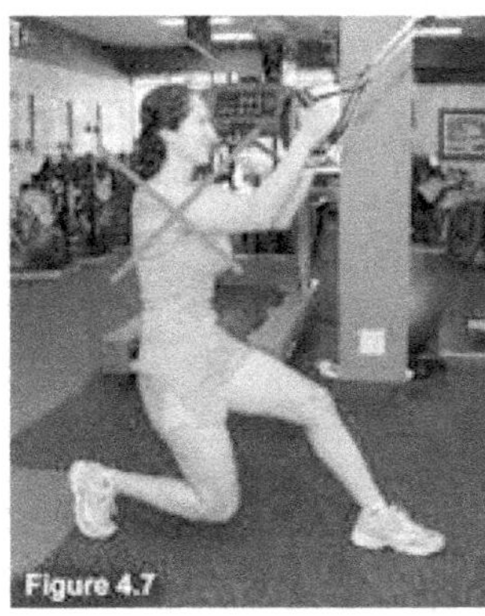
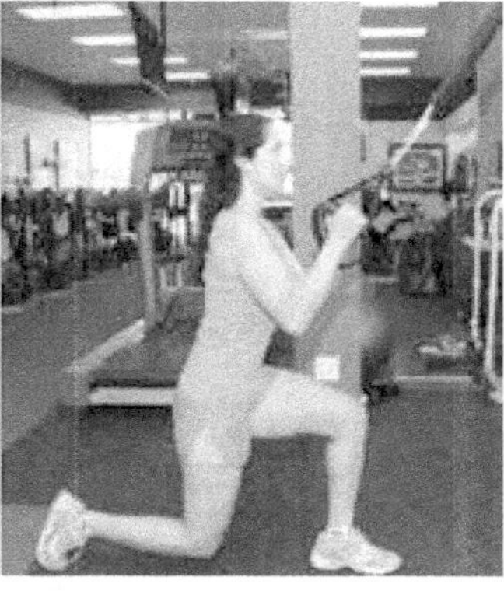

Figure 4.7

Loose Straps: When using a suspended trainer, the straps should always have tension throughout any movement. A common mistake is to allow the straps to lose tension at the top or the bottom of your movement. If you find the straps are loose at any point during the movement, adjust your position to put tension back on them.

Sawing: Keep the straps even at all times. Sawing happens when one arm or leg pulls harder than the other and the strap moves back and forth through the support strap at the top. Most suspended trainers are not made to perform as a pulley. Sawing is not only poor form; it will also wear out your suspended trainer faster.

Now, some suspended trainers, such as the CrossCore®, are made with a pulley rotation device at the top. These are designed for rotation movements with very specific purposes that are beyond the scope of this book. If your suspended trainer includes a pulley system, it should have a locking device that enables it to be used as you would any of the suspended trainers you see in this book.

Conclusion

If you become familiar with what is considered good form, you will go into your movements ready to execute them with the highest quality, get the most from them, and reduce chances of strains or injuries resulting from poor form. This applies to both stretches and strength movements. Once you know what good form feels like, be sure to check in with yourself as you fatigue when performing any of the movements. It's during this time that errors in technique tend to be made. It's also the time when you're giving your body the stimulus it needs to get stronger and fitter. You must teach your muscles to maintain the highest quality of movement execution during this time as well.

Section 2

Strength Training for Stronger Cycling

Chapter 5

Strength Training for Cycling Research

Can Strength Training Really Help Me Be a Better Cyclist?

For some, cycling is a passion and part of who they are. For others, it's just an occasional endeavor for fun, exercise, or to see the world from a different perspective. Whether you enjoy casual rides or hardcore competition, having more strength and stability will result in a more enjoyable ride.

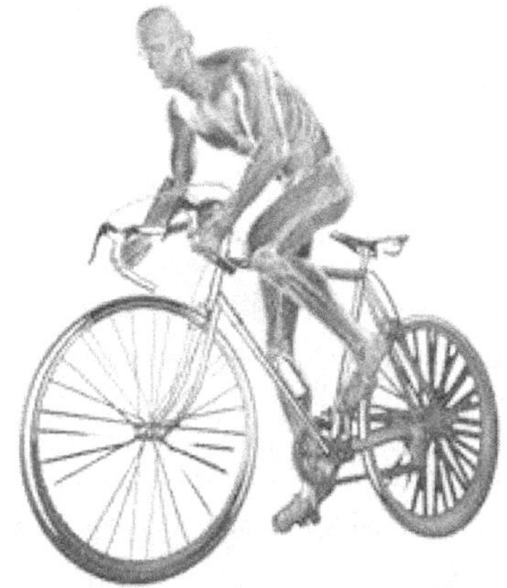

This section will tell you why this is true and how to achieve it through the right approach. I examine details and findings from studies about which aspects of cycling can benefit from performing strength training. For those interested in increasing their cycling abilities through better strength and stability, I also discuss making strength training more specific to the demands of cycling, and more importantly, to the specific type of cycling you do.

The studies discussed in the following section all focus on outdoor cyclists. The experience levels of cyclists as well as the different types of cycling should be considered when performing strength training with the goal of improving your cycling performance. An index of cycling-specific movements that can be performed on a suspended trainer is included in this section for reference. Depending on your level of cycling experience and the type of cycling you're most interested in focusing on, this chapter will help you identify your needs and effectively add strength work to your program.

It is important to mention that information in this chapter is focused on those who participate in outdoor cycling for recreation, health, fun, and competition. Those whose primary form of cardio exercise is spin classes will still get some good insight from this chapter, however, and it would be most appropriate to place themselves in the category of recreational cyclist

What the Studies Say about Strength Training for Cycling

I'll start by reviewing literature on strength training for cycling performance. This section is certainly not required reading, but for some of you, a greater insight will lead to increased yield from workout sessions.

While literature on strength training in cycling is abundant, studies on suspension training and cycling are scarce, as are independent studies of suspension training itself. Most published studies in my review used traditional methods, such as back squats and leg presses, for their strength training programs. I have also attempted to identify studies that use body-weight exercises, or exercises similar to some of the suspension training exercises. Many of the studies compare a control group utilizing a cycling-only training program to an experimental group using the same cycling program in conjunction with a resistance-training program.

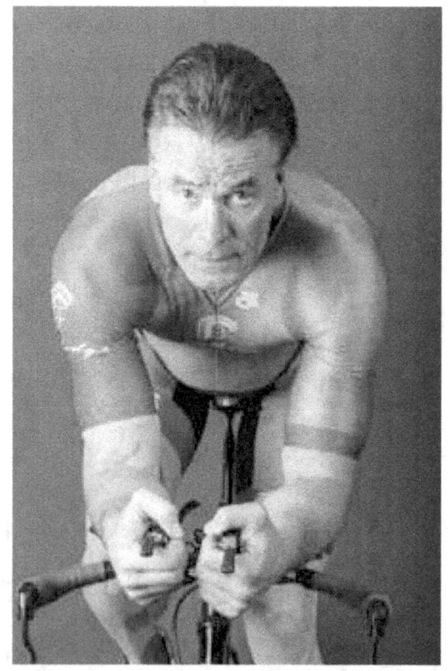

Coming from a weight-training background, I was not surprised to see that a majority of the studies support resistance training as a supplement to cycling performance. Yet it was exciting to note just how many different positive performance adaptations come from resistance training.

Resistance Training and Road-Cycling Performance Studies

Let's start with a review of five independent studies that added a strength training program to cycling training. This was published in the *Journal of Strength and Conditioning Research* in 2010.1 The studies in this review consisted of different strength exercises, populations, and cycling-training programs but tied things together with a common goal of looking at effects on cycling performance with the addition of a strength training program.

In this review, three of the five studies observed significant performance benefits. These three replaced a portion of the athletes' cycling training with resistance training in the control group2,4,6 versus piling resistance on top of the existing cycling program. Additionally, two of the three studies that showed benefits employed high- intensity, explosive-type resistance exercises versus traditional sets of moderately paced repetitions.

The remaining two studies did not show significant performance benefits. Both used traditional, non- cycling-specific strength exercises, such as back squats, leg presses, and machine hamstring curls. Both programs also added resistance-training work on top of existing cycling regimens.3,5 The study in the review which I found to be most relevant to the competitive cyclist, combined both explosive training and high-resistance interval training to the programs of already trained competitive cyclists.2

Previous studies have shown explosive resistance training provides performance benefits, but most of these studies were done during non-competitive season phases. Just one was performed during the competitive season. It combined explosive step-ups with on- bike interval sets of thirty seconds on and thirty seconds off, and it showed impressive results. Performance gains were demonstrated in peak power, which is the highest amount of power they could produce, as well as the average power during both a one-kilometer and four-kilometer maximal effort test. There were also decreases in how much oxygen was needed at a given workload.

Based on this review, you could conclude the following:

1. ***Replacing a portion of cycling training with resistance training while keeping overall training volume static, may be more beneficial than merely adding resistance training to an existing program***. This is great news for time-pressed amateur cyclists. Adding quality strength training is shown to be beneficial for cycling performance, and extending training time to include it is unnecessary. More is not always better (the type A's out there should pay attention). Increasing both volume and intensity of workouts by adding strength work to already challenging cycling regimens, creates a higher risk of fatigue or overtraining, which may cancel any gains. So, cyclists may find reducing their cycling time to add a little strength work is worth the trade-off in performance benefits.

2. ***Explosive movements replicating cycling action are more likely to produce on-bike gains than non-specific exercises***. Weight training is typically symmetrical, whereas cycling is not. In cycling, the rider pushes down with one leg while pulling up, or at least unweighting, with the other. And it's the same for the arms. Add in the associated work of muscles in and around the pelvis, spine, and shoulders, and symmetrical weight training begins to have less relevance to cycling's overall body movement patterns. The study that combined strength training with a cycling regimen in the form of explosive single-leg step-ups (similar to sprinter starts), recorded significant gains, whereas the two studies that assigned movements of primary symmetrical, non-body-weight(such as leg press or back squat) movements did not show significant results.

Results from More Studies on the Effects of Strength Training
on Cycling Performance

Pedal Efficiency Increases. This study on cycling, strength training, and pedaling efficiency compared two groups of cyclists over twenty-five weeks.[7] One group performed heavy strength training; the other did not. The strength training program used included a

> *"It is likely that replacing a portion of a cyclist's endurance training with resistance training can result in improved time trial performance and maximal power."*

squat movement plus two single-leg and hip movements. The group that strength-trained showed more improvement at the end of the twenty-five weeks than the group that did not. The total training time between the two groups was kept equal during the program. The greater improvements in a forty-kilometer individual time trial (ITT) performance in the strength training group were attributed to peak force occurring earlier in the pedal stroke.

Strength Can Be Maintained with Fewer Sessions. The same pedaling efficiency study also supported this idea. The initial ten weeks required twice-weekly sessions with heavy resistance and multiple sets of several lifting exercises. Afterward, sessions were reduced to once every seven to ten days withslightly reduced resistance. Not only did the strength training group experience greater strength gains and performance improvements in peak power, but their mean power during a forty-kilometer ITT was also greater than the control group's after fifteen more weeks of the less-frequent and less-intense program (twenty-five weeks total). This supports the approach that once additional strength is gained, it can be maintained with fewer, less-intense sessions, allowing focus to turn to other training aspects.

Upper Body Strength Matters. Another study looked at results in cycling performance after adding upper body strength work.[8] Force applied to handlebars during starting, climbing, and sprinting, as well as force transfer through the trunk to the pedals, was enhanced by an increase in upper body and core strength. Greater rigidity in the core also translates into more efficient transfer of arm and shoulder forces to the legs during pedaling action. Hill climbs and other strenuous exertions, such as attempting to stay with the peloton or opening a gap on other cyclists, highlight the improvement. Often the moments that matter the most, occur when trying to stay or open a gap with other riders. The extra power you can generate through the core and upper body might just make or break your desired outcome.

Additional Considerations

Without continuing to go into detail on the results of every study out there (which would make this a very long book), I want to highlight some general trends in the literature. These are adaptations that you might experience with the addition of some strength work.

Greater oxygen economy was often observed in a steady-state cycling effort after adding strength training. Applied to you, this would mean your body would need less oxygen at a given workload. This would make you more efficient at producing the same amount of work, which allows you to save energy for later in the race, or perhaps for the running portion of a triathlon. It may also give you the ability to push harder and go faster in any particular effort than you could before, because now you have that extra reserve.

A greater maximum strength of your muscles results in a smaller percent of the muscle's max strength having to be used with each pedal stroke to obtain the same force. This again allows for less demand on your body during the same workload.

Positive adaptations in neuromuscular activation and rate of force development. Strength training is a high-intensity activity that requires your neuromuscular system to learn to use its strongest muscle fibers, and more of them. Your muscles learning how to fire more fibers, and at a faster rate, can result in more power when sprinting, climbing, accelerating out of corners, or catching or leaving behind a competitor.

Conclusion of Research Section

I hope you now understand why strength training should be included in your program. I also hope you now have more incentive to do it. We learned that you don't need to add extra time or a multitude of exercises to your training program. You do, however, need to put a little thought into your program design if you want to achieve cycling-specific benefits from strength training. Although studies on suspension training and cycling were basically nonexistent at the time of writing this book, there were enough body-weight movements included in cycling-specific studies to support the benefits of including this type of strength training in your program. Since suspension training is body-weight training, I think it's fair to assume, for the purpose of designing a strength training program to improve cycling abilities, that suspension training is an acceptable (if not ideal) mode of strength training.

So how do you add strength training to your cycling program in the way that is most effective for you? Your level of cycling, cycling goals, and cycling discipline are all things to consider. The next section will get into more detail on how to select cycling-specific movements and will lay out the best program for you as an individual.

Chapter 6

Bone Health and Cycling

Cycling has a variety of health benefits and is definitely a good activity for your body. However, the research has shown that it does not help create strong bones. In fact, it may even decrease your bone density, depending on the amount of cycling training you do. So, if your sole form of exercise is cycling, you may end up with weaker bones than someone who is not even active! The good news is that you can counteract this with some cross training and strength training.

I also feel that it's important to mention that information in this section is focused on those who participate in outdoor cycling for fitness and competition. Those whose primary form of cardio exercise is "spin" type classes, will still get some good insight from this chapter, but they are less likely to spend extended amounts of time on the bike, and may be at less risk than a cyclist training ten to twenty hours a week. Having said that, bone health is important for everyone, and it's still a good idea to consider it in your fitness program.

Why isn't cycling good for my bones?

There is a lot of research available on bone health and some specific investigations on cycling and bone health. Studies have consistently found several reasons why cyclists have lower-than-normal bone densities...

Cycling is a non-weight-bearing activity. The primary reason for cyclists having low bone density is that it's not a weight-bearing activity. High-level cycling in particular has been shown to have negative effects on bone strength because of the amount of time cyclists spend training and riding. Cyclists spend lot of time seated with no compression forces on the spine and pelvis. Even though it may feel like you are pedaling hard at times, the forces you are putting into the pedals are also not distributed in a way that puts significant strain on your bones, which is needed for bone growth.

Recovery time also non–weight bearing. The necessary recovery time from hard cycling usually involves additional non-weight-bearing activity of sitting or lying down. Most cyclists reported avoiding weight-bearing activities during recovery periods as a way to help enhance recovery from training.

Cyclists generally have lower body mass. Cyclists generally are lighter, and low body mass is another risk factor for osteoporosis and osteopenia. This especially applies to women, who in general have lower body mass, as well as to performance cyclists, who are consistently striving to obtain a low body weight in order to improve performance.

Cyclists have an increased risk of fracture due to crashes or falls. Whether you compete or just ride for fitness and fun, chances are at some point you will take a fall or be involved in a crash. This applies to any level cyclist, whether you ride solo, with friends, in groups, or compete in rallies and races.

Level of Cycling Experience and Bone-Density Risks

If you are a road cyclist, especially if you train hard or have been training for multiple years, you are more likely to develop osteopenia or osteoporosis than the average person. This puts you at a higher risk for fractures, a risk that continues to go up with age and training. In one study, more Masters-Age cyclists were classified

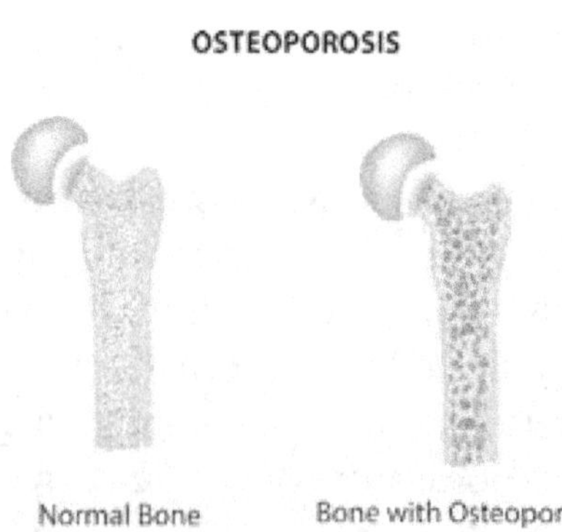

as osteoporotic when compared to age-matched non-athletes, and the percentage of those with osteoporosis or osteopenia, increased significantly after a seven-year period.[10] So for those of you in this category (which may be the majority of people reading this), you are not only more likely to be at risk, but the risk factor also gets higher as you get older, and complete more years of cycling training.

In 2012, there was an extensive review of thirty-one studies on the subject of cycling and bone health.[11] The findings showed that adult road cyclists who train regularly have significantly lower bone mineral density in key regions. This was found to be true when comparing cyclists to control populations of both athletes in other sports, as well as non-athletes. Areas of the lumbar spine, pelvic and hip regions and femoral neck were all key areas found to have lower values in road cyclists than in the control groups with which they were compared.

Included in this review were only a few studies involving amateur cyclists or low-level cyclists (versus more experienced and elite cyclists). Differences in bone mass were not found between the cyclists and controls when compared with low-level cyclists. However, studies that examined elite cyclists, or those training at high levels for numerous years, consistently found low bone mineral density. This further supports the idea that the level of training and length of training are strong factors in cyclists being at risk for low bone density.

Junior Cyclists

Most of the research on differences in bone health considered those older than seventeen years of age. It's worth saying that it's believed that cycling in the early years of life does not negatively affect the bones. However, it doesn't positively affect the bones either. Participation in other sports has been shown to positively affect bone growth more than cycling. Translation: allow juniors to train hard and train often, but make sure they are getting some cross training as well to create maximum bone growth.

Differences Found with Different Cycling Disciplines

Road cycling at a competitive level might be more detrimental for bone health than mountain biking and recreational forms of cycling. This is due to all the reasons stated previously: long hours on the bike, non-weight-bearing activity, no impact forces, low forces in general while pedaling, and lots of time off your feet trying to recover from training.

Mountain bikers were found to have higher bone mineral density than road cyclists. One reason given for this was the vibrations endured during off-road riding. Depending on the level of mountain biking, the increased short durations of high force to get over obstacles may also help.

Sprint-trained cyclists have stronger bones than distance-trained cyclists. This makes sense because of the large forces they generate for short periods of time. The leg muscles are creating high forces, which in turn puts high forces on the bones to which they are connected. The high forces for short durations are similar to the demands of weightlifting. However, keep in mind that this is still a non-weight-bearing activity, so as hard as you might go as a sprinter, compression forces on the spine are still not present.

Triathletes and Duathletes do not appear to experience the same negative effects as those who do only cycling training. The combination of cycling and running appears to counteract the negative effects on bone mass that may result from cycling alone.

Improving Bone Density in Cyclists

Research repeatedly recommends that cycling as a form of exercise should be complemented with cross training and strength training activities to stimulate bone growth. It was also found that cyclists who started weight training and/or plyometric exercises during the long-term studies lost significantly less bone mass. Running has been shown to be beneficial as well due to the impact forces involved. However, both short and long-distance runners will still benefit from including strength work to support overall bone health in their training programs. This is especially true if you have low body weight and run or ride long distances in your training (or both), which requires more nutritional resources. Long-distance cyclists in particular should take heed and be sure to include strength and cross-training activities that put higher forces on the muscles and bones to keep them strong.

We all want strong bones that are resistant to breaking, especially as we age. This is even more important for a cyclist. Let's face it, a crash or fall at some point in your cycling life is likely to happen. Stacking the odds in your favor by including activities to maintain and stimulate bone strength is your best line of defense against a fracture just in case you do happen to hit the ground at a greater impact than you would like.

Put Forces on Your Bones to Make Them Stronger

The aspects that account for bone strength include bone mineral density, content, bone size, and thickness. When muscles contract, they pull on the bones to which they are connected. These forces provide the stimulus for bones to grow both thicker and denser. Maximal strength training and impact forces are the best way to provide this stimulus to your bones. A bone needs to experience a tenth of the amount of force required to break it, in order to be adequately stimulated so it can create increased bone density.[3] Remember this key factor in your strength work.

Don't be afraid to lift relatively heavy weights and add some plyometrics and impact to your program. Jumping rope, box jumps, or even punching a bag for fun provide some impact for your upper body. Adding these elements to your program after developing a foundation will ensure that you are ready for the higher forces these often place on the body (refer to chapter 5).

Strength training results in your body's ability to actually increase the amount of muscle fibers being fired when asked to, as well as how fast they are able to fire. Both of these processes result in the muscles being capable of producing more force, which in turn means more forces exerted on the bones to which they are attached.

In addition to providing greater forces to stimulate bone growth, strength training also reduces risk factors that result in broken bones, by increasing muscle mass and improving balance. This is especially important in older populations of any activity level. If you have better balance, more strength and muscle, and stronger bones, they work synergistically to make you more physically resilient and stable.

You will be better prepared to handle unexpected events, like when your excited puppy darts between your legs, or an unseen slick patch of ground. Your increased athleticism will reduce the chance of falling in scenarios such as these and more. If it happens that you do take a fall, your bones are less likely to fracture from the impact. That's two ways of staying off the injury list.

How to Strength Train for Strong Bones

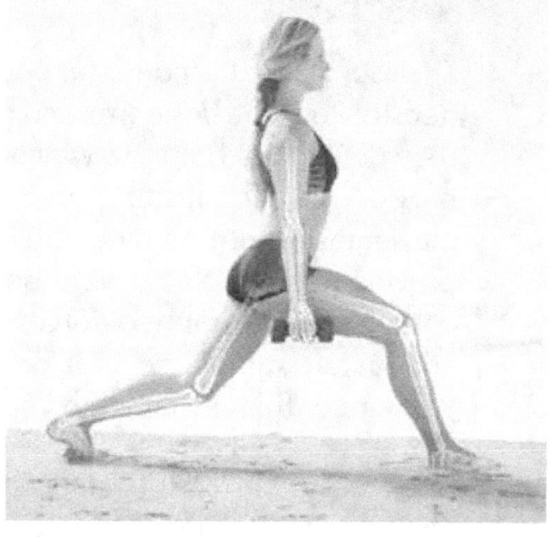

Put random forces on your bones to stimulate growth. Some research has shown that the best results in the short term come out of subjecting bones to high forces in a more random fashion.[4] Shorter-term training programs of more random high-intensity forces on your muscles and bones have actually been shown to be more effective than programs that progress over time. Now, this is contradictory to a program you might put together for performance gain, but it's still something that should be considered if you're concerned about improving bone strength.

Also, these suggestions are based on short-term results. It doesn't mean you shouldn't periodize your program, it's just that in that case, longer periods may be needed to produce the benefits to bone density. If you are following a periodized program and want to make sure it addresses your bone health, my suggestion is to continue along with what you've begun. However, make sure to include one or two exercises that target bone health regardless of what the overall program goals are. The purpose of these movements is to provide the forces on your bones to stimulate adaptation.

Select exercises that involve large muscle groups. The movements involving the larger muscles or multiple muscle groups are all good choices, assuming an adequate amount of resistance is used. This is because the larger muscles can produce more force than the smaller ones. Multiple muscles working together will also be able to generate more total forces on the bones, as well as provide forces in multiple planes of motion.

Allow for longer rest periods between sets to allow for greater force production. Circuit training is a type of training program where individuals perform movements, one right after the other, with little rest, and then repeat the circuit multiple times. It has not been found to be as effective for bone and muscle growth as a program with longer rest periods and higher resistances. Because the short or absent rest periods in a circuit program don't allow for recovery, the forces you can push are lower. Circuit training may still help with bone health in the long term and is still great exercise. However, if stronger bones are your goal, design a program that involves more strength, higher forces, and longer rest intervals. This will allow for more maximal forces to be produced during the sets.

If you are someone who likes to attend group circuit classes or who is not as comfortable lifting heavy weights or pushing with high force, you should be aware that you are at greater risk for osteoporosis. In addition, if you are a cyclist or long-distance runner who doesn't utilize strength training or doesn't lift heavy weights for whatever reason, you are also at risk. This is particularly the case for lighter and leaner individuals.

Choose movements to load key areas of the body. The results of multiple studies reveal that bone density is site specific. This means that all of the bicep curls and chest presses in the world will not help you increase bone density in your hips and pelvis, as much as doing lower-body movements that put stress on the hips and pelvis. Lumbar spine stress is achieved by loading weight on the back and spine, such as doing deadlifts or squats with weight (done with proper form) and by performing sit- up-type movements and back extensions. Stress on the femur occurs when legs are put under heavy load or impact forces. Thus, if you want strong bones in your hips, legs, and spine, make sure you include resistance movements that target those areas. Conversely, if you have a particular region of the body you are concerned about, be sure to give that area some more love with additional site-specific exercises.

Include jumping, sprinting, and plyometrics in your program.
Impact movments and movements in which loading is applied at a high rate also provide more stimulus for bone growth. This includes jumping, sprinting and plyometic activities. [5] in addition, if you participate in sports such as tennis, basketball, or other activities that involve jumping, accelerating, or quick changes of direction, you have a definite advantage when it comes to maintaining strong bones. Saying this, devleoping a foundation of strength(chapter 5) in these movements before progressing to more intense jumping and sprinting activities is crucial to ensure

your muscles and tendons can handle these high and changing directional forces.

Beyond suspended training. In addition to suspended-training movements, consider adding movements where the spine is placed under load, such as squats with a bag, bar, or a standing machine. Loading up a leg press might be beneficial for the hips, but it will not put the necessary compression forces on the spine needed to stimulate bone growth. The "farmer's walk" (an exercise where you are simply carrying heavy weights); pressing; pulling or lifting heavy kettlebells or dumbbells; barbell work; kicking, punching, or flipping heavy bags; jump roping; pull-ups; high-intensity running, shuffling, or cutting; and jumping are all good additions that will stimulate bone growth. These can supplement your suspended-training program if you have access to additional equipment. An example of this would be performing a suspended squat jump followed by a suspended push-up with high resistance, and a sprint to the end of the block. These would be three extremely beneficial exercises to stimulate bone growth.

Conclusion

If you are concerned about your bone health, it doesn't mean you need to turn your program upside down. Simply include one or two random exercises that stress your legs, hips, and lumbar spine with some impact and force. If you are just starting to strength train or know that you already have low bone density or osteoporosis, the more explosive exercises should be phased in gradually as you improve your strength and fitness level. Always develop the foundation before adding higher intensity or more specific work to your program. Just keep in mind that being consistent and including bone-building activity in your program during the long term, will produce benefits.

Chapter 7

Developing a Strong Foundation

This is the most important chapter of the book when it comes to developing a solid foundation of strength and stabilty that will support your running demands. This chapter will give you the tools to help you put together a training program and improve overall strength at your level. It will also give you a foundation of fitness that will set you up for success when progressing your program to more run specific strength movements.

I will go over why it's important to consider your long-term goals and what you want to get out of your training program. This will prevent you from making the mistake of jumping into a random collage of workouts, repeating the same workout for too long, or running out of ideas to keep you engaged and progressing, which can cause you to gradually lose interest. A suspended trainer is the only tool required for designing workouts using this book, with any fitness objective in mind. However, it's not mandatory that you use suspension training for all exercises, and it's not necessary that you limit yourself to only suspension training if you have the resources to include other types of training.

Designing a medium-term or long-term program is not necessary to start training. However, it can give you direction and help you progress properly toward your medium and long-term goals. It can also help you stay on track and hold yourself accountable. With that said, the structured approach may work better for some than for others. If your style is more on the unstructured side, this is still the best place to start out, and you may still find yourself returning to this section as your fitness level advances.

What Is Periodization?

Having spent time in the personal training world, I have too often come across people who exercise consistently but have reached a permanent plateau. The most common scenario is that they have been stuck on the same program for months or even years—the same exercises, same repetition ranges, and same amounts of resistance. Their bodies have already adapted to the program and are not getting any overload or demands that require any more change. Whether you are a performance-oriented endurance athlete or someone who wants to lose weight and obtain better general fitness, the way to do that is to continually challenge your body with new demands. In a variety of studies, periodization has been shown to result in more fitness gains.[1]

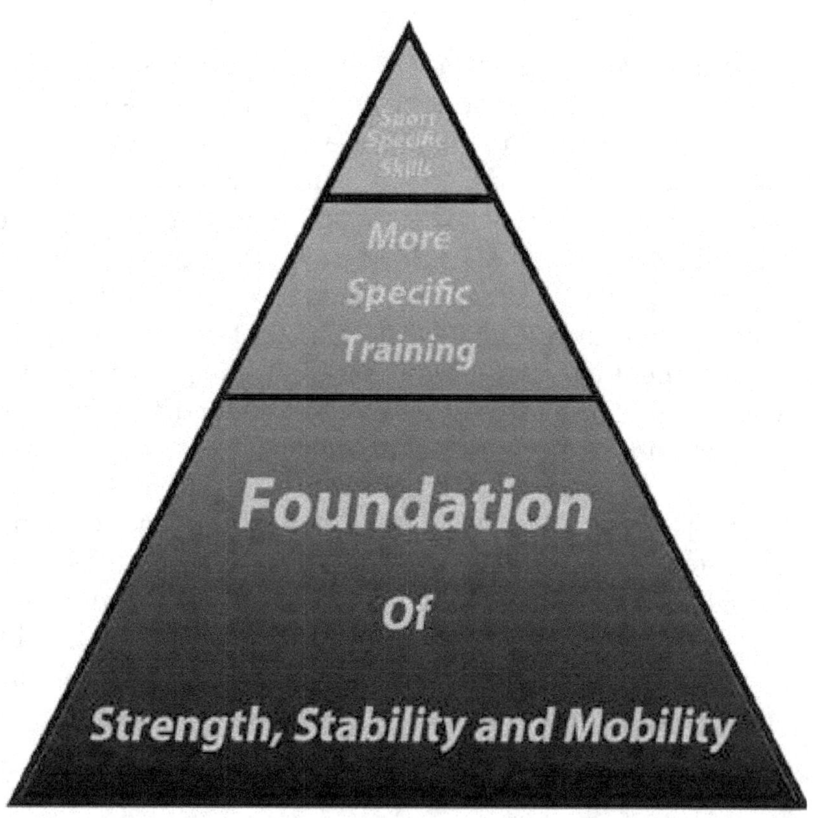

weight loss. Finally, a competitive runner might transition from a general strength program, to a strength maintenance program, to coincide with a structured run training program.

Periodizing your training into phases or blocks that will keep your body working harder and adapting to new demands, while getting adequate rest to recover and rebuild, is the route to continuing improvement. If you are a competitive runner, you may already be applying these concepts to your run training program. We are going to take the same approach to your strength training.

Generally, each phase has certain objectives, and you work on targeting things during your workouts that will best result in you meeting those objectives. The following chapters go into further detail on a variety of aspects, such as cardio, strength, performance for running, or bone density, that you may want to focus on during a training phase. These phases may build on one another, focusing on just one aspect at a time, or they may shift in focus to completely distinct aspects.

Periodization can be done within a block of training. The simplest approach would be to focus on increasing the amount of resistance you can move at a targeted repetition range. You

> **Periodization:** *Conditioning programs can use periodization to break up the program into phases or training blocks. Each block has specific aspects and goals on which it will focus. A phase can be built on the work achieved during the phaswe preceding it, or it can shift focus to a different objective.*

could also reverse this and aim to increase the repetitions you can perform at a given resistance. Another approach might be to increase the number of sets or duration of work intervals over the course of a block of training.

Periodization can be done over the span of several blocks of training. A traditional approach would be shifting from using sets of lower resistance and higher repetitions in one training phase, to sets of higher resistance and lower repetitions in the next training phase. Another example would be a recreational runner, designing a six-week training plan to focus on general strength, followed by a six-week training program to focus on cardio and

For instance, if you are interested in targeting more cardiovascular benefits or are pressed for time, it would be beneficial to plan a four-to-six-week block of workouts that include movements which use multiple muscle groups and/or have short, or no, rest periods between sets. If you are concerned about osteoporosis and want to improve bone density, you could choose exercises that work large muscle groups with high resistance, or exercises that involve some impact. If you are combining suspension training with other methods, you have limitless options when it comes to program design.

DON'T SKIP OVER THIS SECTION, ESPECIALLY IF YOU ARE NOT ALREADY INCLUDING RESISTANCE TRAINING IN YOUR PROGRAM!

I cannot stress this enough. Even if you are a seasoned runner, strength training will challenge your muscles with movement patterns and intensities they will have to adapt to. Treat your training program like building your dream house. Make sure the foundation is solid to achieve a high quality of the overall program and to avoid cracks developing later as you transition to more specific movement.

After you have obtained a general ability and comfort level performing movements on a suspended trainer, you should start thinking about your goals for the next training block. You may want to plan your upcoming phases by choosing to alter any number of variables, depending on your goals or preferences, with the goal being to improve on those aspects and keep your program dynamic and effective.

hings you can change within a workout:

- movements performed

- the number of sets performed

- the number of repetitions performed

- doing sets of repetitions versus time-based sets

- the level of resistance

- the rest between sets

- the number of exercises

- the speed at which you perform the exercises

Things you can target within a training phase:

- building a solid foundation

- building strength

- gaining muscle

- improving cardiovascular health

- targeting weight loss

- improving balance and stability

- improving flexibility

- improving bone density

- sport-specific strength

Start Your Program Off Right

A solid foundation to your fitness program is not unlike a solid foundation to your house. It may not always be the sexiest part of the program, but it's the most important building block. If you want to be able to perform advanced progressions or intensity, a solid foundation will provide necessary support, and you will be more likely to handle the higher intensities and complex movement demands. However, adding intense training on top of a weak or cracked foundation may result in bad technique, less efficient workouts, or even breakdown and injury.

To build your foundation, start with a general all-around workout that targets multiple movements and challenges strength, endurance, and stability. Maintain balance in your exercise selections by including movements that counter each other. For example, employ a pushing movement and a pulling movement that work opposing muscle groups, like push vs pull. Another example evem more specific to running is to master a basic split stance movement, squat movement and hip hinge movement in your intial foundation phase. These movements will develop leg and hip strength, and stabilty that are important for a solid run stride. Select basic movements and perform them at a comfortably challenging resistance level. I recommend a repetition range of about 15 reps per set during this phase. This will give you a moderate degree of resistance and enough reps to develop muscle memory and coordination of the movement.

The unstable platform of the straps is something your body may not be used to, and this will allow it time to learn the most efficient muscle-firing patterns, as well as stabilizer recruitment of the muscles involved. I also suggest an initial block of at least four to six weeks to develop this. If you are new to strength training, make that six to eight weeks, and consider doing more than one training block of foundation work. Everyone will have his or her own level of experience, ability, and comfort. If you don't have much experience strength training, a longer block of time or multiple training blocks of foundation work will allow for your strength, balance, coordination, flexibility, and overall kinesthetic awareness to further develop.

You may experience improvements during this time, as you become comfortable with the movements. Many of these initial gains will be neuromuscular as the body becomes more efficient and figures out which muscles to turn off and which ones to activate. The neuromuscular system is a quick learner. The structural components of your muscle fibers, tendons, and ligaments take a little longer to catch up and adapt to the new demands being placed them. Be patient, and give them the chance to do so.

You may still periodize within this phase, over multiple foundation blocks, by progressing the movements. Your ultimate goal should be improving all-around strength and stability. As you get stronger, you should be able to advance in movement progressions or in the resistance utilized for each given movement selected.

Getting Started with Your Program

A good start would be to choose one movement from the beginner exercise library that can be found at the end of this book, each focusing on a different movement pattern.

- pushing
- pulling
- legs and hips
- core

Once you've completed this phase, and have achieved an adequate comfort and ability level with a program of basic movements, you may want to change things up. This may involve simply continuing to build on that foundation with a modification of the exercises you select. Changing or progressing the movements performed, while keeping the repetitions, sets, and rest periods the same will accomplish that. You may also want to shift the focus to strength, cardio, or a sport-specific strength program.

Sample Workout to Get You Started

At the end of this book is level 1 beginners foundation workout and a level 2 intermediate foundation workout to get you started. The goal of the program is to get you comfortable and more experienced using the suspended trainer, and to develop an initial foundation of improved strength and stability.

Conclusion

Start your training off right with the recommendations in this chapter.

You will achieve a balanced program with movements that complement each other. You will also develop a strong foundation of strength and stability. You will be able to build on this and transition to more run specific movements, and/or a maintence program as you ramp of the intensity of your run training depending on your season or chosen events.

Progress at your own pace. Don't worry about what exercises others may be doing. Find the exercise, progression, and resistance level that are right for you and your goals within that workout. It should be challenging to finish each set while performing the targeted number of repetitions. You should also be able to complete the targeted number of repetitions without changes to form or a reduction in the range of motion. Don't move to the next progression or more advanced movement until you have mastered the current one.

Consider all the variables you can manipulate within each workout and each training phase. You may change any of these variables to target your fitness goals, choosen running events, or simply to keep things interesting and prevent plateaus in your fitness. Periodization to your program can be done over weeks, months, or even years.

Consistency is key. Stick with it.

Chapter 8

Making Strength Training Cycling Specific

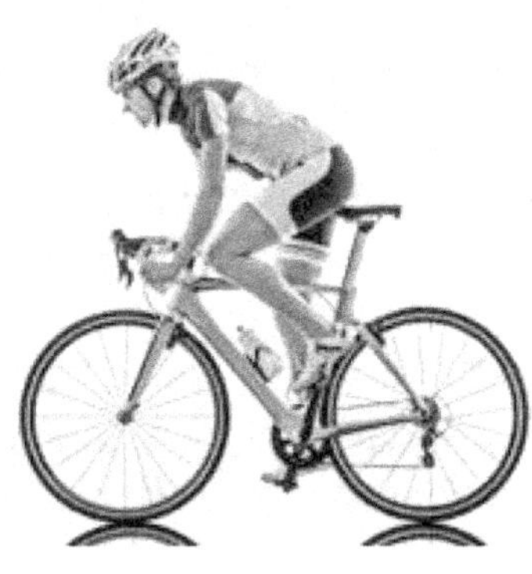

The SAID principle is a widely known and accepted principle in athletics. SAID stands for "Specific Adaptations to Imposed Demands," and it basically means that your body will adapt to the demands placed on it in the same way that those demands are placed on it. It's pretty simple. If you train with a lot of fast and short intervals, you will develop speed. If you ride for long durations at a slower pace, that is the focus upon which you will be adept. The same thing applies to strength training.

Knowing this, select movements can be included that are relevant to cycling.

Basic cycling demands include:

- Generating power through the legs and hips

- Legs working in sync but independently

- Balance

- Adequate mobility of the hips and torso

- Power transfer from the upper body to the lower body through the core

- Control of both internal and external factors through the core

There are additional, more specific demands if you're focusing on a specific cycling discipline, and I will cover those shortly.

The following is a list of suspension training movements that are specifically beneficial to cycling. This list is designed to give you some choices when putting together your own program. **Level 1** movements are more basic and offer a good place to start for beginners. These can be progressed as you get stronger and your abilities develop.

Level 2 movements are more advanced and/or complex movements. These are merely suggestions on good movements that are relevant to the demands of cycling, so don't feel like you need to limit yourself to only these, or even to only suspension training. Give some thought to what movements in general are most relevant to cycling, or to the type of cyclist you are. Focus on your specific goals, and apply them to all methods of resistance training you choose to use. The next sections talk more about things to consider based on both your ability level, and the type of cycling discipline in which you participate.

Level 1 Movements

- Bicycle Kicks
- Plank
- Split Squat
- Reverse Lunge
- Hip Hinge
- Push-Up (Hands Suspended)
- Row
- Half-Kneeling Roll-out
- Half Get-Up
- Suspended Get-Up
- Sprinter Starts
- Hip Raises
- Triceps Extensions

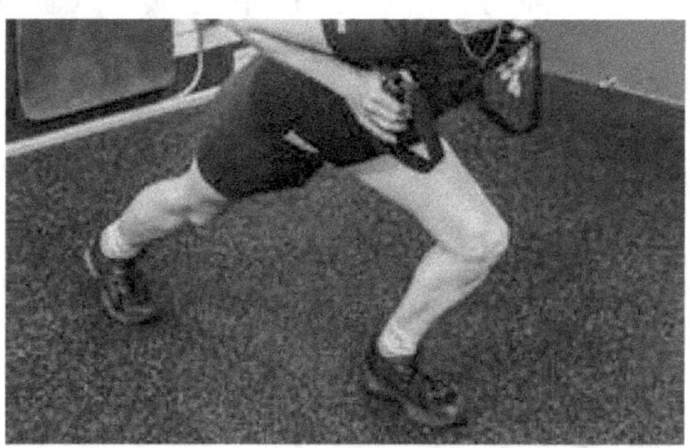

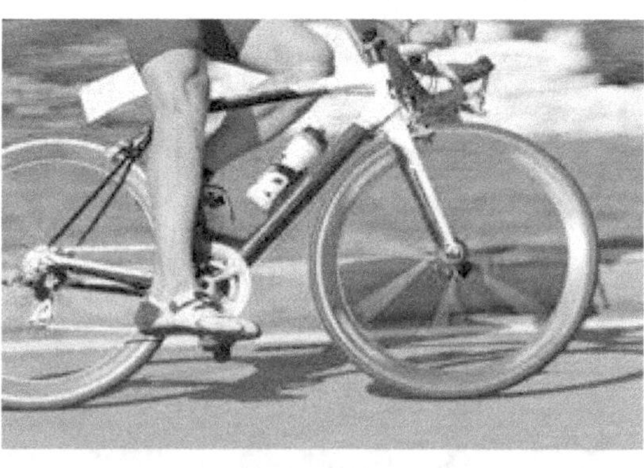

Level 2 Movements

- Single-Leg Squat
- Suspended Reverse Lunge
- Suspended Power Lunge
- Push-Up (Feet Suspended)
- Atomic Crunches
- Mountain Climbers
- Suspended Side Plank
- Tall Kneeling Roll-out
- Inverted Row
- Pull-Ups or Assisted Suspended Pull-Ups
- Overhead Squat

Although all the suspension training movements listed in this section are cycling specific, not every exercise will yield maximum benefit to every cyclist. This is because different types of cyclists have different sets of demands on their bodies. They are also coming from different levels of fitness and ability. A recreational cyclist may need to increase overall strength and stability to allow for more comfortable and enjoyable rides, while a track cyclist may need a program for increased power development. The first thing to consider is…what type of cyclist are you?

Three broad types of cyclists are covered in this book: recreational, fitness, and competitive. Each of these requires its own level of fitness and has demands specific to that discipline. Each may also attract individuals with much different levels of ability and exercise experience. Suspension training can play a part in helping all three of these types of cyclists achieve their goals.

No matter what category a cyclist falls into, he or she will benefit from a solid general foundation of strength and stability. Building that foundation during the first block of a strength training program is crucial, and this is true for all categories of cyclists, from beginner to elite. The level 1 or 2 foundation workouts are a good place to start for anyone who is beginning a strength program for the first time or someone coming back to strength training after a break.

Recreational and Fitness Cyclists

Cycling experience and objectives:	Areas to work on:
Beginner-level cyclists Cycling for enjoyment Cycling for exercise Improving cyclist	Stability in gusting crosswinds Handling unexpected obstacles Maintenance of correct posture Increasing comfort on the bike Reducing fatigue to enjoy the ride longer

You want to have fun on your bike, feel healthy and strong, and enjoy being out in the open air. Maybe you're getting into cycling for the first time, or maybe you have been riding for years. Most cyclists in this group have no desire to keep pace with anyone other than for good company. It's sufficient to feel strong on your bike and complete a ride without becoming unduly fatigued. This category may include beginner or intermediate-level cyclists and exercisers.

Developing a strong torso and core will delay the onset of fatigue and provide assistance if fatigue does set in. This requirement applies very much to cycling, where controlled pelvic movement is at the center of the activity. Fatigue and loss of posture may cause discomfort along the spine in the lower back due to lack of conditioning in the muscles supporting the stomach, spine, and pelvis—in other words, lack of core strength. Additionally, working on correct movement patterns will help maintain good mechanics during pedal stroke, and increase endurance levels when the rider is confronted with a steep hill…or when turning a corner and realizing the tailwind that was such a friend on the first part of the ride is suddenly an adversary.

Comfort is crucial. If you are not comfortable on your bike, it's not going to be enjoyable. A proper bike fit is important for this aspect. Adequate mobility in your own body is equally important. It supports greater comfort during rides and can prevent excessive physical strain due to riding position.

Fitness and Fast Recreational Cyclists

Cycling experience and objectives:	Areas to work on:
Intermediate-level cyclist Experienced cyclist Cyclists who ride with a group and in rallies Former racing cyclist who rides strong but no longer has specific competition demands	Stability in gusting crosswinds Handling unexpected obstacles Maintenance of correct posture Maintenance of efficient pedal stroke Increasing power and speed Lowering overall fatigue

You ride hard and like to push yourself. It's important to you to keep up with your riding buddies and groups, and to survive tough hills, surges, periods of high pace, and long rides or rallies. You want the same increased strength and stability as a recreational rider, but you may already have a higher level of fitness thanks to your more intensive training. This category may also include seasoned cyclists who are not training at competition level in terms of structure, volume, or intensity.

You don't have to worry as much about specific demands and periods of competition as a competitive cyclist does, but you would still benefit from building up your abilities on a suspended trainer to the more advanced progressions and movements.

Designing a Program for Recreational and Fitness Cyclists

Recreational and fitness cyclists generally benefit most by selecting exercises that emphasize building a foundation appropriate to their ability levels. Make it a priority to focus on form and proper progression of the difficulty level because:

1. Recreational cyclists may be coming from a beginner's fitness and ability level, and would benefit most from developing functional strength and balance to support their cycling.

2. Fitness cyclists may have a strong level of fitness, but lack a history of strength training.

3. The fitness cyclist who has a high level of both cycling fitness and strength training may progress quickly to the more advanced movements, but will always benefit from the basics.

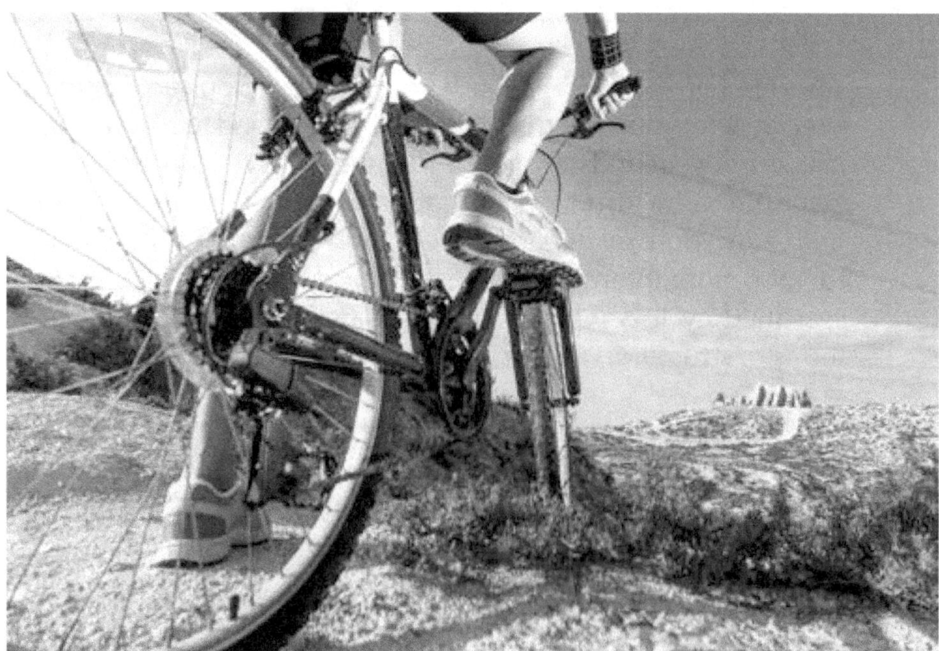

Competitive Cyclists

Cycling experience and objectives:	Areas to work on:
High level of cycling fitness Currently in competition or training to compete Focused on a specific cycling discipline Riding with fast groups and pacelines (road or track) Training solo with specific goals Usually follows a structured regular training plan	Rapid accelerations and force generation Stability in gusting crosswinds Handling unexpected obstacles Targeting specific demands of the discipline Maintenance of efficient pedal stroke Fatigue resistance under high intensities Obtaining high power numbers specific to the discipline

Competitive cyclists train hard to be able to perform at their best for specific types of events. They need to consider the demands of their events as well as have an overall plan that will have them riding strongest when it matters most.

Subcategories of competitive cyclists include off-road, triathlon, mountain, track, and cyclo-cross. Each of these disciplines requires a solid foundation of strength and stability, and has a specific set of demands.

Any suspension exercise under the recreational and fitness categories will also benefit competitive cyclists in any sub-discipline. I highly recommend beginning a strength training program by following the recommendations found in chapter 5 or by selecting from the exercises detailed later in this book and mastering, at minimum, a three to four week program. During this initial block, focus on mastering the technique and progressing the difficultly level of each exercise. Stick with the same movements, but vary the difficulty level as you get stronger. This will also allow adaptation to training demands on a neuromuscular level as well as develop the strength and structure in your muscle tissues necessary to handle the demands of more advanced movements that will come later.

Competitive cyclists with a strong fitness background will be more likely to progress to more advanced exercises and progressions. Many are more complex and require more stability and strength, while some are plyometric in nature. Following are a few things to consider for each discipline when selecting exercises to augment an already established program.

Triathletes. Top priorities are mobility and fatigue resistance. Triathletes need a strong, stable, and fatigue-resistant pedal stroke. They also have to maintain an aerodynamic position on the bike for extended periods of time. Transitioning from the bike to running with efficient mechanics, requires optimal mobility from muscles that may have been in a shortened position during the bike leg.

The need for short bursts of acceleration for a few seconds at a time is also beneficial for gaining momentum out of corners and passing competitors within the time allowance. Think about choosing movements that develop the core and upper body to hold the aero position, as well as to train the hip, knee, and ankle to remain in alignment during both the pedal stroke and single-leg run stance.

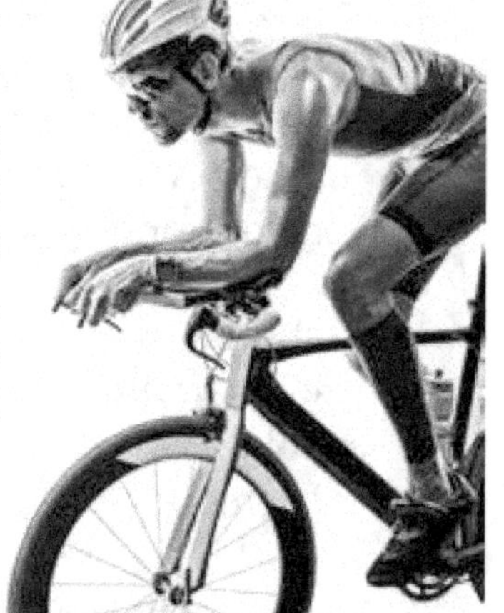

Include some stretches to ensure adequate mobility in all areas.

Road. Top priorities here are fatigue resistance and overall strength and stability. Racers need to maintain a solid, efficient pedal stroke through repeated anaerobic efforts and adverse conditions.

A strong torso is crucial for providing a solid center to transfer force to the pedals during accelerations, climbing, and sprinting. Upper body strength is part of this strong center and can help with the push-pull dynamics that generate transfer force to the pedals in climbing and sprinting. Think about 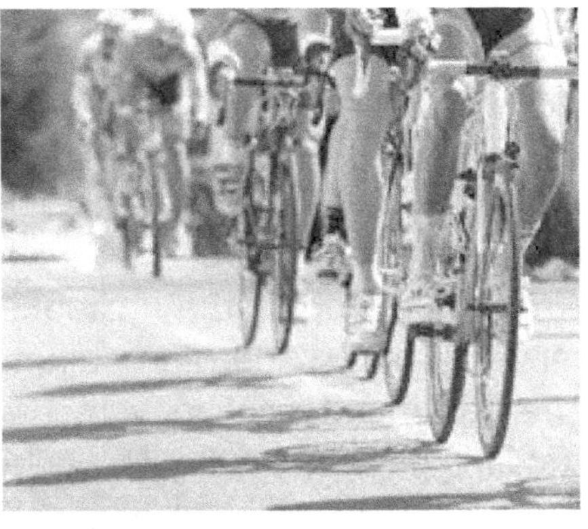 choosing movements that develop stability of the hips, knees, and ankles, as well as movements that require full-body strength where the core stabilizes through the center.

Track. Top priorities are power and repeatability of short, hard efforts at high speeds. The demands of track racing include activating as many muscle fibers as possible, as fast as possible to create maximum acceleration as soon as possible. Track cyclists need to be able to repeat multiple short, hard sprints with periods of high-threshold intensity in-between. They also need a very high leg speed to achieve high cadences while producing large amounts of force.

Choose exercises that emphasize power development and have an explosive or plyometric component to them. These exercises will develop the neuromuscular systems as well as the large-muscle fibers that are responsible for quickly generating high amounts of force.

Mountain. Top priorities are stability and repeatability of short, hard efforts. Mountain bikers need full-body strength and stability to control the bike on rough terrain. They also need strength and proper alignment in their pedal stroke across a wide range of RPMs.

The hand position during mountain biking is pronated, which is different from the other disciplines, and is something to think about mimicking when selecting exercises to develop strength through the wrist and arms.

Mountain bikers often need to be able to lift up the front of the bike while stabilizing the back of the bike. This requirement of having strength on top of the unstable platform of the bike on rough terrain makes suspension training ideal for developing strength. The platform of many movements on a suspended trainer is a very similar type of instability. Upper body, core, and full-body strength can be developed to also handle extreme instability during the strength movement. Choose full-body movements that involve the core stabilizing through the center. Progress to single-leg movements that require force generation and stability during hip and knee extension and flexion. Some work on unstable surfaces may also benefit this discipline.

Cyclo-cross. Top priorities are overall stability, mobility, and repeatability of hard efforts. This discipline requires a variety of demands. CX riders need strength in their pedal stroke, as well as strong torsos to transfer force and control the bike on adverse terrain.

Cyclo-cross often requires lifting up the front of the bike over obstacles or dismounting and carrying the entire bike while running (often over soft and unstable ground), climbing, or hurdling barriers. A strong core that can handle asymmetrical loads is crucial. Running up steep inclines, over barriers, or through sand pits requires hip and knee stability and fatigue resistance. In addition, adequate hip mobility is needed for hurdling barriers and remounting the bike.

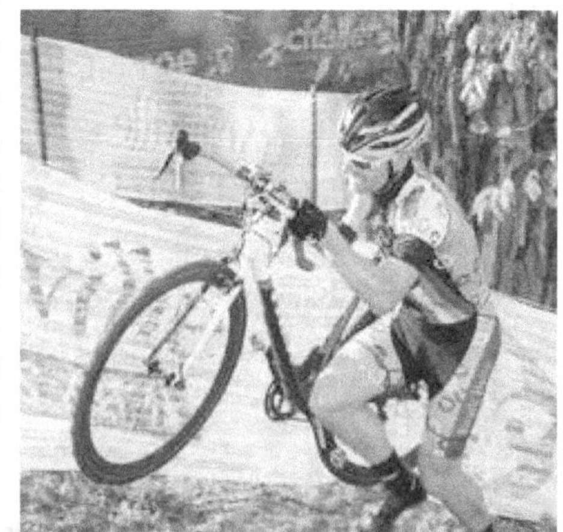

Choose full-body movements that involve core stabilization and transfer of power through the center of mass, and single-leg movements that require explosive extension and hip stabilization. Also include some upper body and core exercises that require the body to move or stabilize with one side only.

Ultradistance. This may include ultradistance racing or long-distance touring. Fatigue resistance and comfort on the bike over extreme durations of time, are your top priorities. Proper pedaling biomechanics and core stamina are also extremely important and must be maintained for long durations of time.

Choose both dynamic and static stretches to make sure you have adequate mobility of the ankles, hips, torso, and upper body. Choose core as well as full-body movements that require stabilization and power transfer through the core.

Sidebar: A Cautionary Note for Competitive Cyclists

This chapter assumes you are at a high level of fitness and ability. Thus, some advanced suspension exercises are included, and these require high levels of body awareness, strength, and stability. If you are a racing cyclist but not yet skilled in suspension training, ease your way in. One of the biggest mistakes I see is people who immediately jump into the most advanced exercises when starting a suspension-training program. Some of these individuals can just about manage the movements but usually have incorrect form and are unable to execute the full range of the movement.

It's a bit like doing anaerobic intervals on the bike before you've established your endurance base. Not only will you not achieve your potential, but compensations occurring to complete the movement can likely result in negative forces on the body.

No matter what your cycling level is, I strongly recommend you start with the intermediate movements and progress to the advanced movements when your skill level allows for it.

Designing a Program for Competitive Cyclists

If you are a competitive cyclist, you probably have a training plan that focuses on a racing season. Even if you don't race, there are still times of year that are better for cycling no matter where you live. You may want to be at your best fitness for a cycling trip or particular rally.

The *Hotter'N Hell Hundred* is the largest sanctioned century bicycle ride in the country and takes place in Wichita Falls, Texas, in August. Too many times I've had clients who want to start training for this or other similar events but start too late in the game, and end up paying the price on event day (and sometimes for weeks after).

There isn't really a time not to resistance train. However, if you have a structured plan, there may be an optimal way to select what exercises to do, and incorporate them into your training schedule.

Off-season or preseason is the time when most cyclists start thinking about strength work. One of my goals in writing this book is to help more people actually perform strength work to supplement their cycling, as well as to make it easier to include in their training plans. For those who are not really sure what to do in terms of strength training, I have given a little direction below to refer to when planning your workout. If you're following a plan targeting one or a series of competition events, the basic rule is as follows:

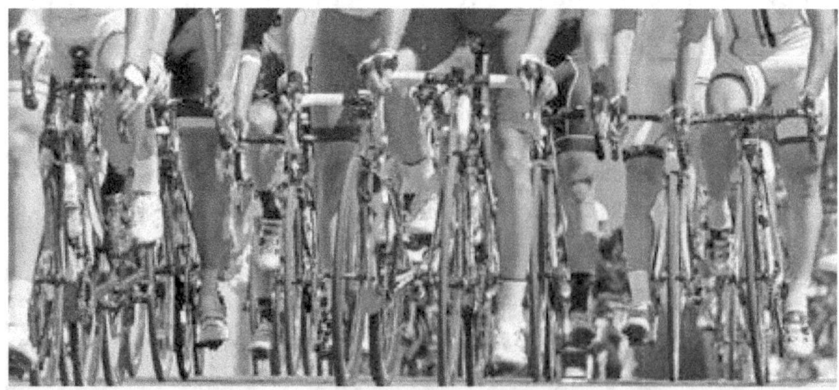

General>Specific> Maintenance

Start with a general program to give you a chance to build a foundation and master the movements. After that, get more specific with the movements you're selecting and executing, and consider the demands required by your type of cycling. As you approach your event or the peak of your competition season, transition into a maintenance program you can use on a more infrequent basis. This allows for the majority of focus to be on competition events, or on-bike training sessions, while maintaining the strength and stability obtained.

Preseason Program

This is a more generalized program that will give you a foundation of strength and stability, as well as more comfort with using the suspension trainer. The strength and control you will develop with this program will create an important foundation necessary to support the next phase. This consists of a balanced program of upper body, lower body, and core movements. Refer to the level 1 and level 2 foundation workouts on pages 212 and 215 for an example of this program. Because the focus is general strength and stability, the workouts are appropriate for a wide range of people who may have different goals and abilities they will be considering after obtaining a strong foundation.

Do this program twice a week for four to six weeks. You may progress during this time by adding resistance, or moving to the next progression for any given movement. However, continue to build on the similar movement patterns. This allows for strength to be built upon the gains made in previous workouts. You may also add a third strength or cross-training workout of your choice, depending on how well you feel you're recovering from the workouts, and what you're doing in addition to your strength program.

Early Season Program

Progress to more difficult exercises, complex movements, or

higher intensity and explosive movements.

Consider the individual demands of your chosen cycling discipline. Is it your priority to develop short-term power, increased stability, or fatigue resistance? Think hard about the things your chosen cycling discipline requires from you when selecting movements, as well as when executing them in your workout. Refer to the previous sections for each discipline to spur some ideas for exercise selection.

Competition Season Maintenance Program

Back off the intensity and focus on stability and maintenance of the strength you developed in the previous program(s). According to the study referenced earlier in this chapter, strength gains can be maintained with a frequency of as little as one session every ten days. In addition, this session need not be of maximum intensity. This will allow you to go into your race-specific intervals, or races themselves, with more freshness, but still with the strength and stability you obtained in the previous training blocks. In this phase, I suggest putting on-bike work first in your program, and focusing on race-specific fitness. Remember, the goal is simply to maintain the strength and stability gains you have made due to the hard work you have done over the last several months.

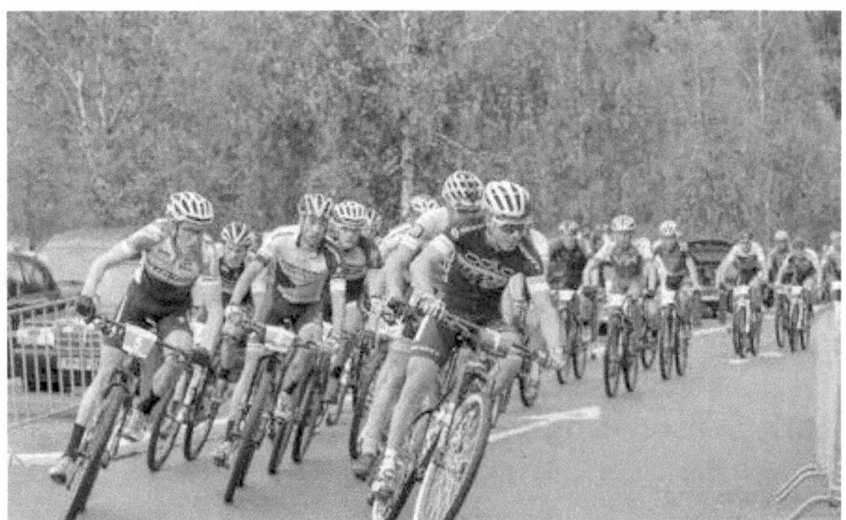

During a taper or the week preceding a key competition event, I suggest leaving strength training out of your program altogether. This will ensure optimal freshness during that event. If you are undergoing a multi-week taper for an endurance event such as an Ironman or ultradistance event, you may want to keep it in until the final week of the taper, but be sure to reduce the intensity and focus on the stability component. Strength training during this time should not leave you too sore, as you should not be increasing the intensity during this time or shifting the types of movements you are doing. Stick with movements you have been doing in the weeks preceding, and remember that the goal of a taper or the week preceding competition is to allow your body to recover and rebuild from previous training.

Chapter 9

Exercise Movement Libraries

The exercise movement libraries in the following section have been divided into Upper Body, Lower Body, Core and Whole-Body movements.

Each section starts off with more basic and beginner friendly movements and progress to and the more intermediate and advanced movements toward the end.

Chapter 9

Upper Body Movements

Lower Body Movements

Core Movements

Whole Body Movements

Golf Rotation   Upper Body

This movement is a great one for loosening and warming up the upper torso and arms. It's also excellent for increasing shoulder and upper-torso mobility for those who are lacking it, and to help open up the chest for easier breathing and improved upper body posture and positioning on the bike. The rotation and reach will also help posture and form by strengthening the muscles in the upper back.

Focus: Upper back and shoulders.
Setup: Straps fully extended.

1. Face the anchor, hold the straps, and get into a shoulder-width stance.
2. Keep one arm in place and reach up and slightly behind you with the other arm, rotating your torso and looking in the same direction.
3. Hold for one to three seconds on each side. Alternate sides.

Those of you who spend a lot of time at a desk or behind the wheel during your day will really benefit from this movement, because it will increase the strength as well as the mobility of your upper torso.

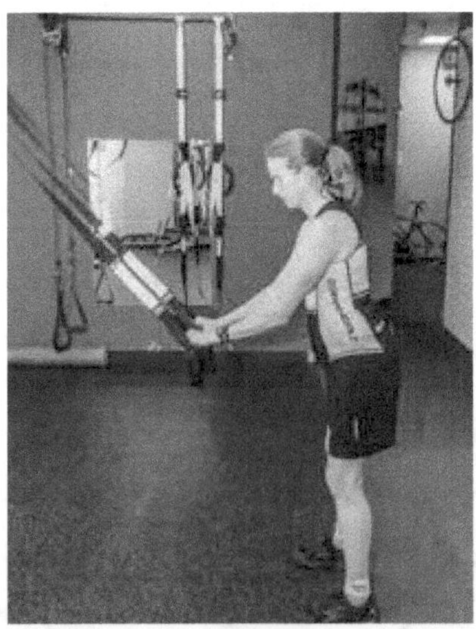
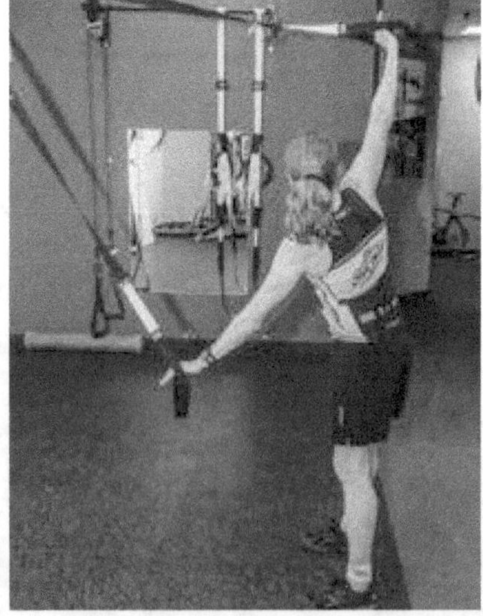

Suspended Push-Up   Upper Body

This is an all-purpose pushing movement that increases both strength and stability of the upper body and core.

Focus: Chest and shoulders.
Setup: Straps fully extended.

1. Face outward, holding the straps with arms straight in front of you.
2. Allow your arms to bend, and lower your body until your elbows reach ninety degrees and are aligned with your shoulders. Don't let your elbows get behind your shoulders.
3. Push yourself back up to the straight-arm position, exhaling as you do so, and maintain a tight core and straight body from head to feet.

Note: Keep your arms up at shoulder level as you descend(don't allow your elbows to drop. Keep your core tight and body straight (don't allow the hips to sag) throughout the movement.

To make it harder, step back to load more of your body weight onto the straps. To make it easier, step forward to load more of your body weight onto your feet

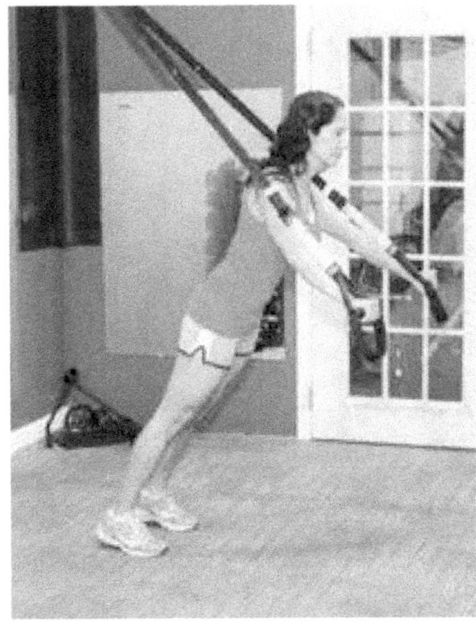
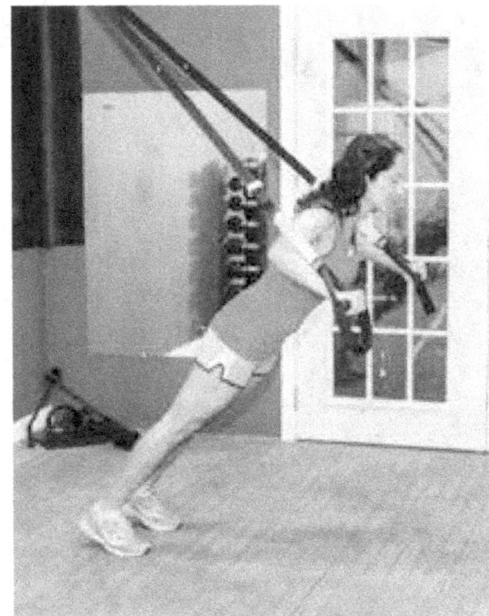

Suspended Row   Upper Body

An all-around movement that targets the large muscle groups in your back. It can improve posture by strengthening the muscles that pull your shoulders back. This move is especially great for those who spend extended amounts of time at a desk, computer, or behind the wheel.

Focus: Back and arms.
Setup: Straps shortened to mid-length.

1. Face the anchor point, holding the straps with a shoulder-width stance. Lean back and straighten your arms.
2. Pull yourself up until your elbows are bent and at your side again, exhaling as you pull yourself up. Keep a solid core and straight body position from your head to feet and your head aligned with the spine.
3. Lower yourself back down by allowing the arms to straighten until you are at the bottom of the movement.

To make it harder, step forward and place your feet farther underneath the anchor. This will increase your lean, putting more body weight on the straps, which is more weight you'll have to lift.

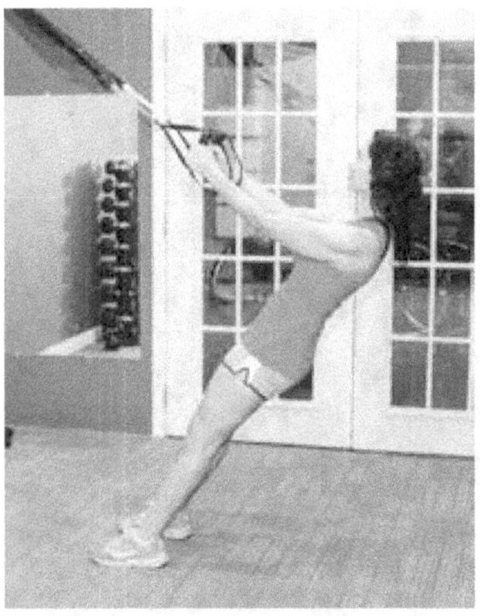
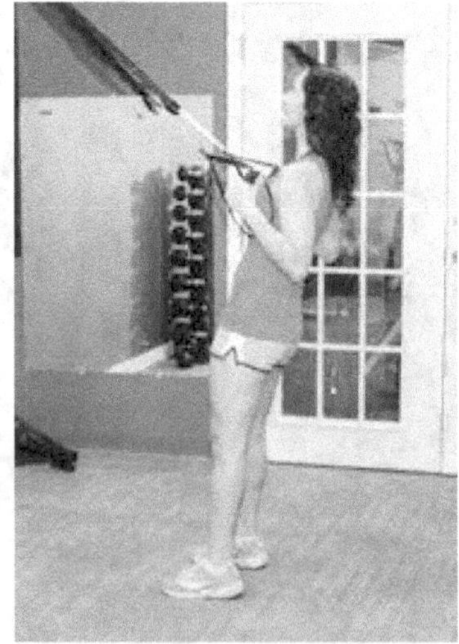

Single-Arm Row Upper Body

A rowing movement with a twist—literally. You are pulling, which strengthens the back muscles, and you are also generating rotational forces through your core. You might want to relate this on e to the push-pull action on the handlebars during hard climbs or sprints.

Focus: Back and arms.
Setup: Straps mid-length and single-handle mode.

1. Face inward, and hold the single handle with one hand. Get into an offset foot stance by stepping back with the foot opposite the hand that is holding the handle.
2. Allow the arm holding the handle to extend, and reach for the floor behind you with the free hand. Allow your weight to shift a bit to your back foot if needed.
3. When you get to the bottom of the movement, pull yourself back up, and finish the rotation by reaching forward with the free hand toward the strap.

To make it easier, get into a wider offset stance, or position yourself more upright so more of your weight is being supported by your legs. Also, although you will rotate your torso and hips, still maintain good posture, and keep your body straight like board.

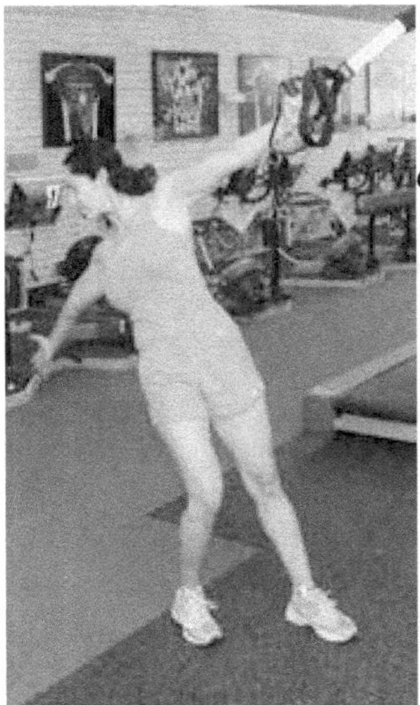
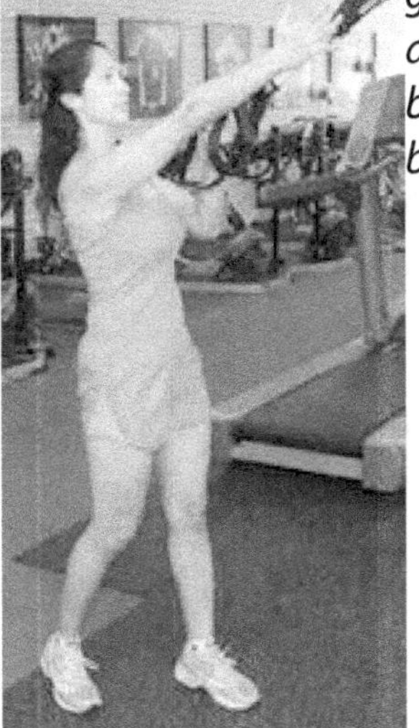

Suspended Pull-Up Upper Body

This is a pull-up that allows you to assist and self-spot by pushing a portion of your body weight with your legs. A great all-purpose pulling movement that makes pull-ups accessible to a variety of strength levels.

Focus: Back and arms.
Setup: Straps super-shortened, which will allow you more room underneath to perform this movement.

1. Start by sitting on the floor directly underneath the suspended trainer, holding the handles, with your knees bent.
2. Pull yourself straight up from the floor and up until your chin is level with your hands. Think about pulling yourself over an imaginary bar.
3. Hold your position at the top for a second with good form and then come back down in a slow, controlled movement. Keep the elbows out wide, shoulders back, and chest out as you're pulling yourself u

Use your legs to spot you as much as you need to but as little as you must. Perform as much of the work as you can by pulling yourself up with your arms

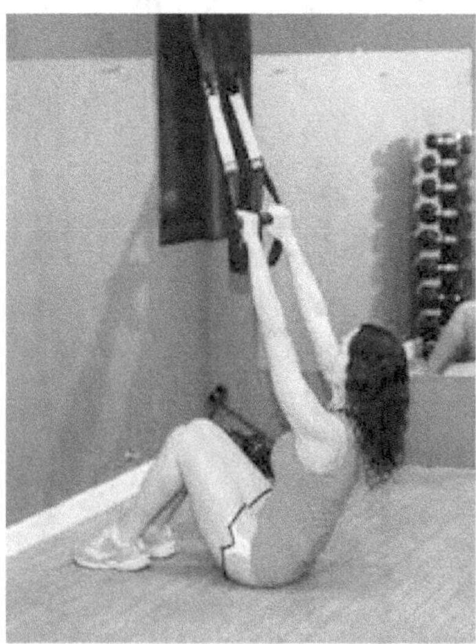
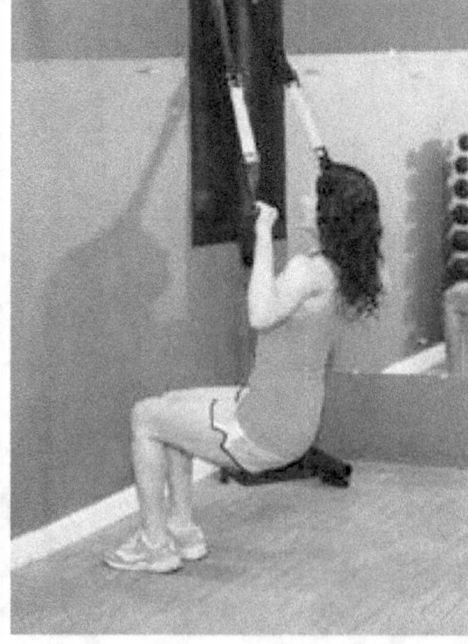

Push-Up with Feet Suspended   Upper Body

A great all-purpose pushing exercise. This version of the push-ing movement requires torso and upper- body strength as well as proper timing of the stabilizer muscles to maintain a straight body.

Focus: Chest and arms.
Setup: Straps fully extended and approximately six to twelve inches off the ground.

1. Face away from the suspended trainer on your hands and knees with your toes in the cradles, right underneath the anchor. Your hands should be slightly wider than shoulder width, and your thumbs should be aligned with your chest.
2. Start by straightening your legs, which will lift your knees off the ground. Keep your body straight, and go down until your elbows bend to approximately a ninety-degree angle.
3. At the bottom, push through the floor to raise your body back up to the starting position as one unit.

Keep your core tight, and don't let your back or hips sag during this exercise. Also, keep the hands inline with the chest. The imaginary line between your hands should be directly under your chest (not your face).

*This version of a push-up should not be attempted until you can perform several full traditional push-ups first. Become proficient with push-ups first by performing push-ups on your knees, or hands sus-pended. Advance to suspending your feet at that point.

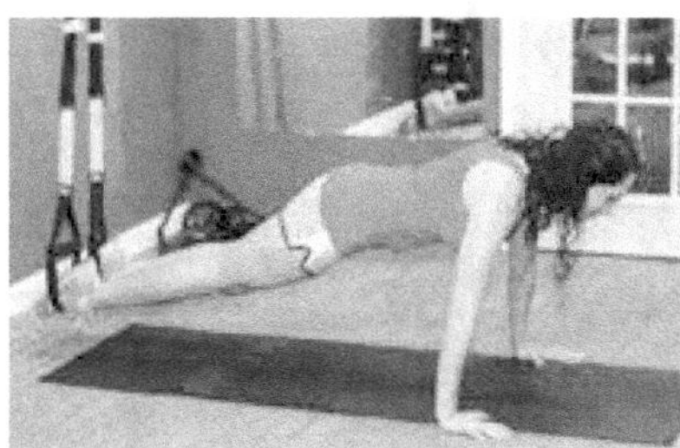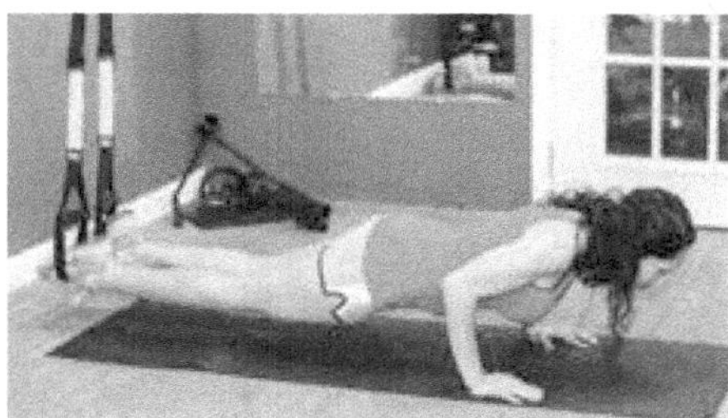

Reverse Fly
Upper Body

This move targets muscles needed for good posture and positioning on the bike. Those of you who spend a lot of time at a desk or behind the wheel during your day, and then bend over your handlebars training in the evenings and weekends, will really benefit from this one because it will strengthen the back muscles that pull the shoulders back to help maintain good posture.

Focus: Upper back and the rear part of the shoulders.
Setup: Straps fully extended.

1. Face the anchor with your arms extended and together in front of you with a slight backward lean. Place your feet in an offset stance with one foot in front and the other foot placed behind you.
2. Keeping the arms straight, open them up, and extend out from your shoulders. This will bring your body forward.
3. Bring the arms back together to the front, holding good form as you do so.

Keep your abs engaged, and do not allow your back to arch as you bring the arms back. This is especially important to remember as you fatigue during the set!

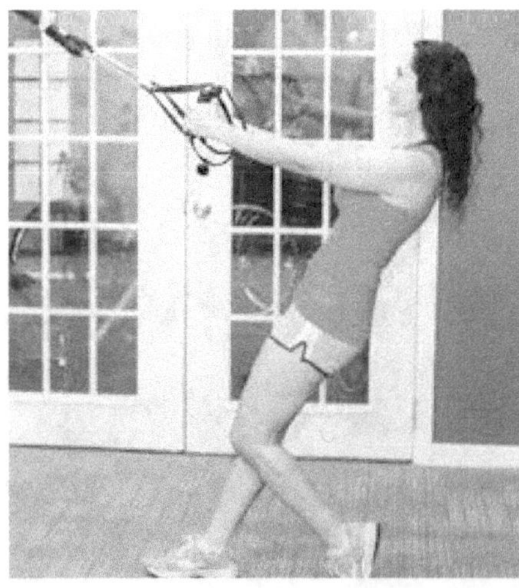
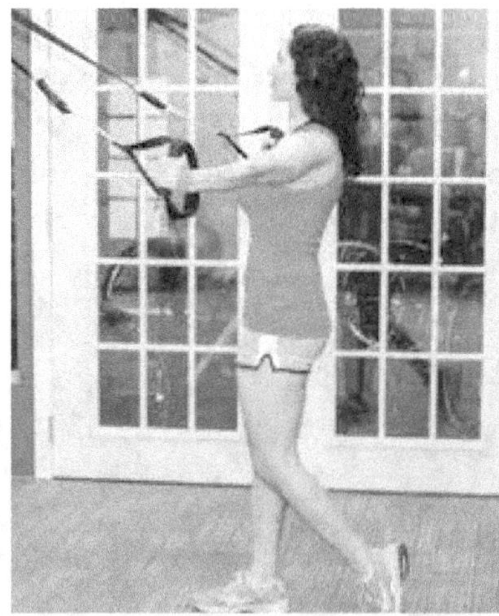

Back Extension　　　　　　　　Upper Body

Since this movement targets the entire back side of the torso and core, it helps develops good posture and a stronger, more injury-resistant torso and may also help in maintaning good posture on and off the bike.

Focus: Back and rear shoulders.
Setup: Straps fully extended.

1. Stand and face toward the anchor, holding the handles.
2. Allow your hips to hinge, and push your butt back behind you while keeping your arms straight.
3. At the bottom of the movement, extend your arms up over your head as you bring your hips back underneath you to straighten your body again.
4. Note: Maintain a strong connection with your shoulders. Think about pulling the shoulder blades in and down toward your pockets.

Performing a seated version will take the hips out of the movement and target the lower and upper back only.
Make sure to extend the arms through the full range of motion

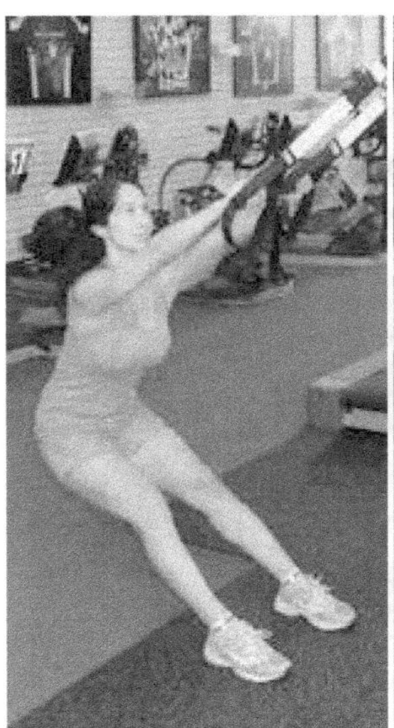
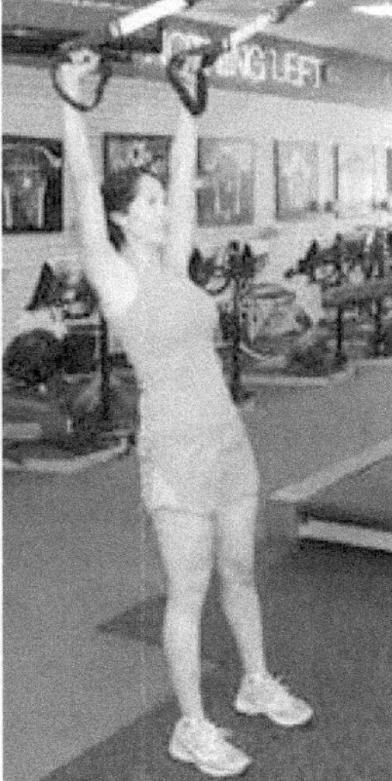
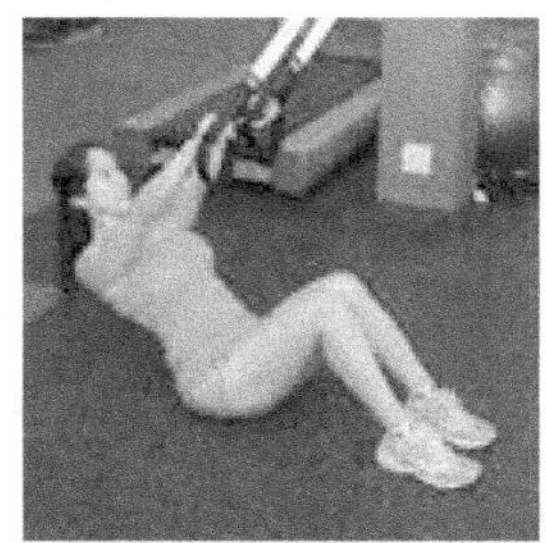
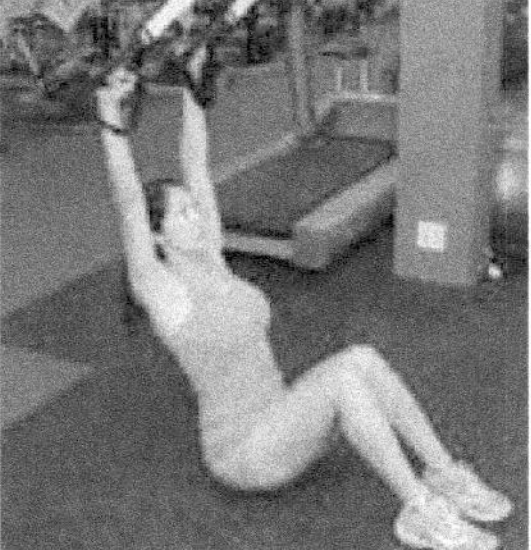

Triceps Extension

This one targets the underside of the arm, and that's where you should feel it. You will also feel this in your core as you maintain your position during the movement. You are basically doing a triceps press and a plank at the same time. This is a great one for triathletes as it strengthens the muscles of the core and upper body that are used to hold the aero position for extended periods of time.

Primary Focus: Triceps.
Setup: Straps fully extended.

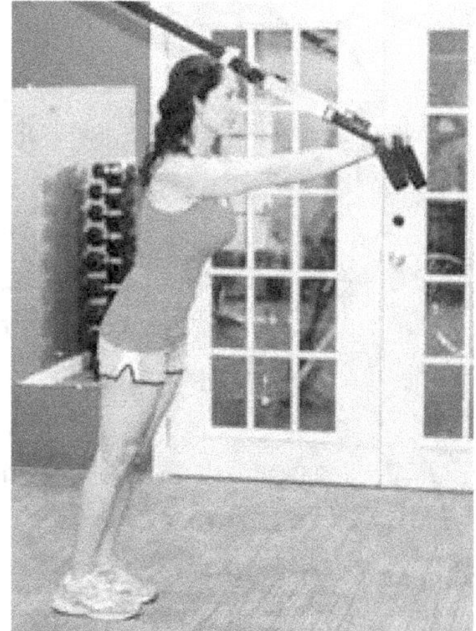

1. Face outward, holding the straps with your arms straight in front of you and parallel with the ground. Start the movement by allowing your elbows to bend and your body to descend toward your hands.

2. Allow your body to come toward your hands until the tops of your hands are close to your forehead. Always maintain your tight core and a body straight like a board.

3. Return to the starting position by straightening the arms and pushing the body back up and away from the hands.

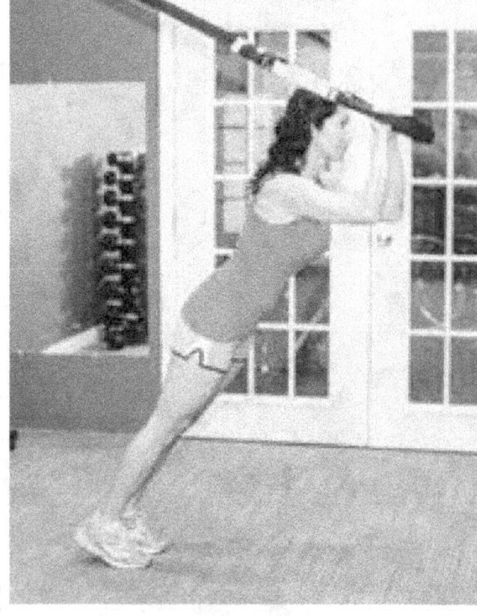

Keep the elbows in and up! Your upper arm from your elbow to shoulder should remain parallel with the ground as your elbows bend. The most common mistake in form for this movement is to allow the elbows to drop or flare out. Keep them high and tight. They should point straight ahead at all times.

Wall Slide

An excellent movement for increasing shoulder and upper-torso mobility, strength in the upper back, and improved posture in all activities. This one is more important for you as a cyclist than you might realize. This is especially true if you have a sedentary day job. If you spend a lot of time either on or off the bike in a seated, leaning forward position, this movement can help counteract that. If is also harder than it looks if you really put the effort into it.

Primary Focus: Upper back and shoulders.

Setup: Straps fully extended.

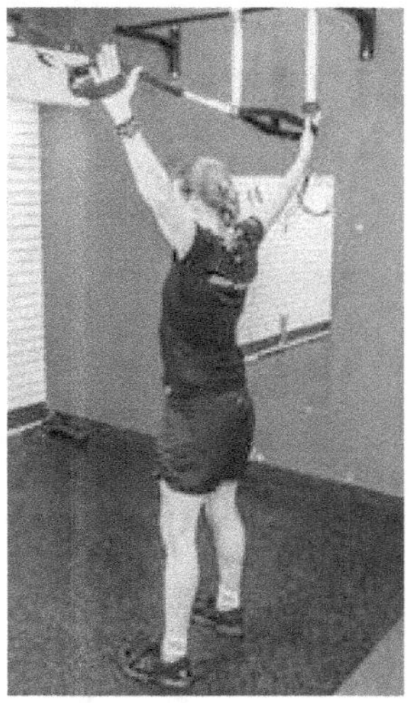

1. Face the anchor with your arms up, elbows bent and at shoulder level, and the backs of your hands pressed into the foot cradles.

2. As you continue to press your hands back into the foot cradles, extend your arms upward until they are completely straightened.

Keep your abs engaged, and do not allow your back to arch as you bring the arms back. This is especially important to remember as you fatigue during the set!

If your hands tend to migrate in front of your body as you press them overhead, you might have some limited mobility in the upper spine and/or shoulder area. Work on this one by focusing on pressing the backs of you hands into the straps and working through the range of motion as much as you can.

Split Squat   Lower Body

This movement develops strength and balance control in the legs and hips. This movement pattern of the legs and hips working together, although they're in opposing positions. It is important for overall good movement abilities, gait mechanics and even applies to pedalling mechanics as you are working the legs and hips in opposition to each other

Primary Focus: Front and back of the legs as well as the hips.
Setup: Straps fully extended or shortened to mid-length.

1. Face the anchor and hold the straps in front of you. Take a large step behind you with one leg while keeping the other leg where it is.
2. Begin the movement by dropping the back knee down toward the floor as low as you are comfortable doing. The knee of the front foot should stay directly over that foot as it bends.
3. Return to the starting position by pushing through the toes of your back foot and the front foot.

Widening your feet will make you more stable. Narrowing your feet will challenge your balance more.

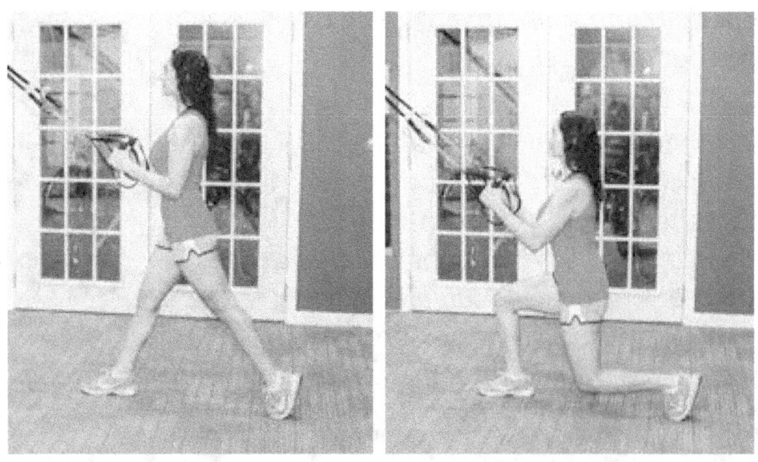

Reverse Lunge   Lower Body

This is a great exercise for your single-leg strength and stability because of the requirement of decelerating, stabilizing, and then pushing your body weight forward with one leg at a time. Training the muscles to not only be strong in a single-leg stance, but also to be stable is a critical component in maintaining strong pedal mechanics especially on climbs, out of the saddle intervals and through fatique.

Primary Focus: Hip and legs.
Setup: Straps fully extended or shortened to mid-length.

1. Face the anchor, holding the straps. Take a big step back with one foot, and immediately drop the back knee straight down to the floor. Descend to a depth that challenges you.
2. From there, ascend by pushing up through the front leg and bringing the back leg back to the starting position.
3. Repeat all repetitions on the one leg, recover, and then perform a set on the other leg.

The front leg is the one you want to be working. Focus on pushing through that leg to return to the starting position from the bottom. The knee should be right over the midfoot as you descend and ascend. If you feel wobbly or your knees tend to cave inward, don't descend as far down, and focus on improving the stability of the

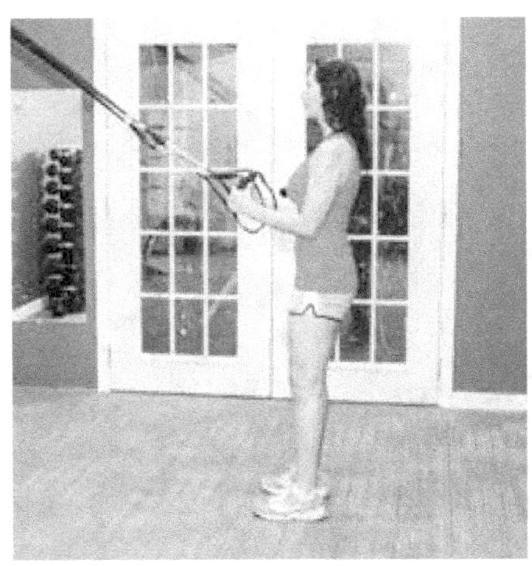 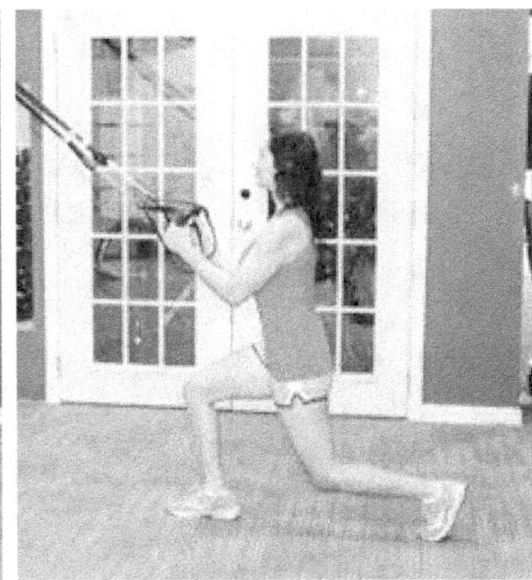

Hip Hinge

Lower Body

This movement will train the muscles to maintain stability while supporting the body on one leg. This is relevant to the pedal stroke in cycling. A lack of stability in your pedal strong can result in lost energy, compensations and even injuries. Even small amounts of lateral movement (such as the knee slightly caving in with each pedal stroke, which is more common than you might think) can add up over thousands of repetitions. I have personally experienced the benefits of this one after developing pain in my adductors and having my cycling coach at the time identify the error in my pedal stroke.

Primary Focus: Legs and hips.
Setup: Straps fully extended.

1. Face the anchor, holding the straps. Lift one leg and extend it behind you while bending forward from the waist and pushing your arms out in front of you.
2. At the bottom of the movement, your body should be as straight as possible from your arms to your extended foot. Think about making a flat table out of your arms, torso, and leg. Maintain a strong, stable position with the supporting leg, with the knee directly over the foot and hips aligned.
3. Return to the starting position with both feet on the ground again. Do not lock out the knee.

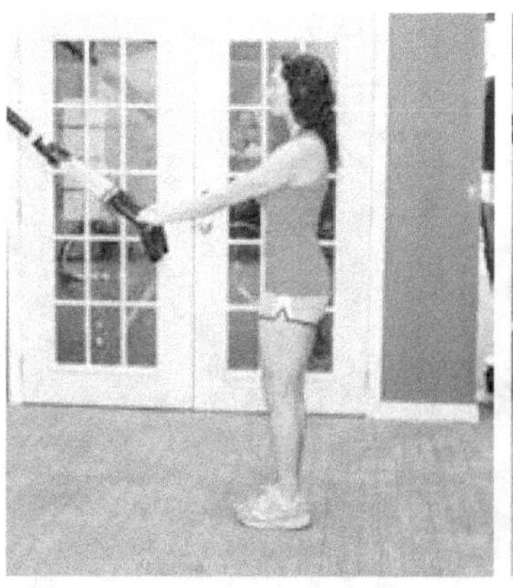
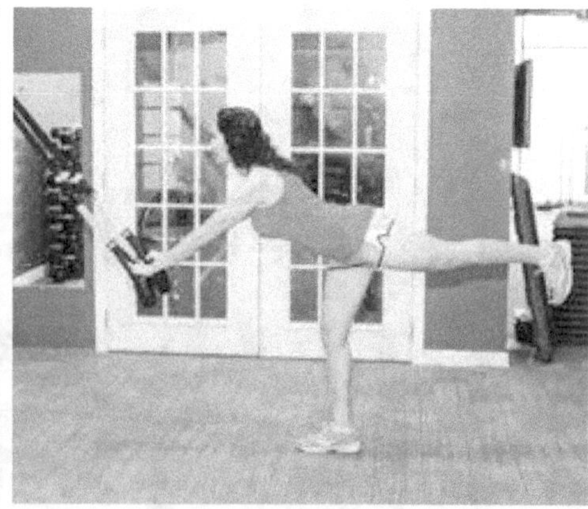

Hamstring Curl

This movement will develop hamstring power and strength that can contribute to the back end of your pedal stroke. This movement, especially in combination with some spin scan sessions, may help to smooth out your pedal stroke.

Elevating your hips during this movement also strengthens the back side of the core. This exercise can also be done as a combination with the hip raise. Instead of keeping your hips elevated, just lower them back down and then lift them back up between each hamstring curl.

Focus: Hamstrings.
Setup: Straps fully extended and six inches off the ground.

1. Lie on your back with your feet in the cradles of the straps and your knees slightly bent.
2. Keeping just a slight bend in the knees, push through your heels and raise your hips.
3. Keep them elevated and pull your heels toward your butt. Extend your legs back out, keeping the hips raised. Repeat.

This movement is harder than it looks. But if you still want more, move your position farther out from underneath the anchor point (see chapter 3 on adjusting resistance levels). You'll be working against gravity more and will have to overcome more resistance to pull your heels to your butt.

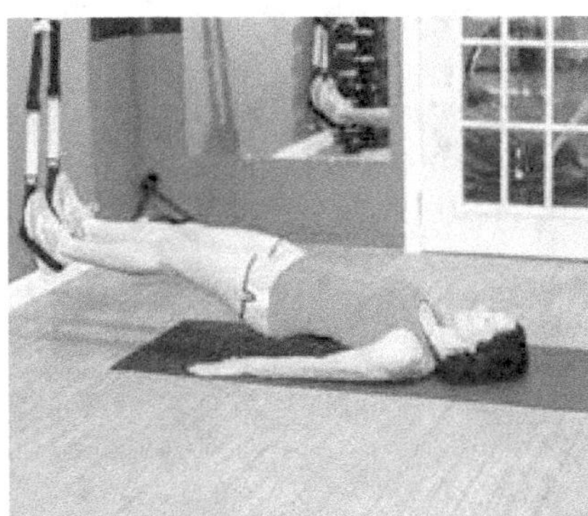 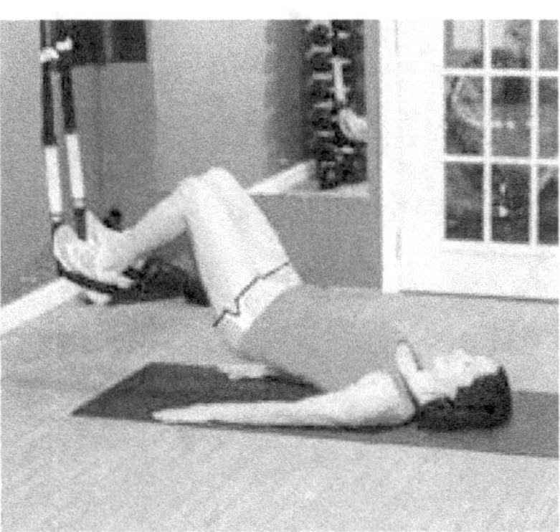

Suspended Front Squat

The squat is an all-purpose movement that will strengthen the legs and hips. It develops strong hip and leg extension. This move can also progress to the front squats with the jump, which is a great exercise for developing explosive power as well.

Focus: Front and back of the legs as well as the hips.
Setup: Straps fully extended.

1. Start by facing away from the anchor with the straps underneath your arms. Place the handles between your thumbs and index fingers with your elbows bent and at your side.
2. Lean into the straps so they're supporting a portion of your weight (think about making chicken wings with your arm and elbow position). It's OK if your heels come off the ground when you're leaning forward, but your body should stay in a straight line. You should feel like you're just hanging on the straps at this point.
3. Allow your knees to bend and your hips to descend back and down behind you toward the floor, following along the angle of your lean.
4. At the bottom of the movement, make sure you still have good posture and a tight core, and push back up, exhaling as you do so. Maintain your torso position (don't bend over at the waist), and look straight ahead (not at the floor).

Start slowly and increase the speed of the movement as you become more comfortable. Add a calf raise at the top of the movement for more bang.

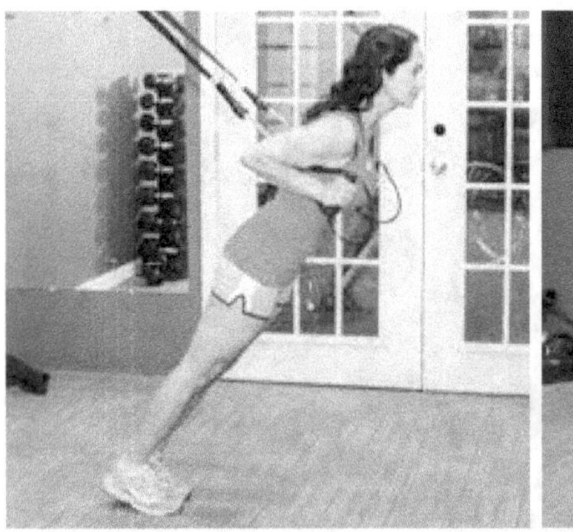
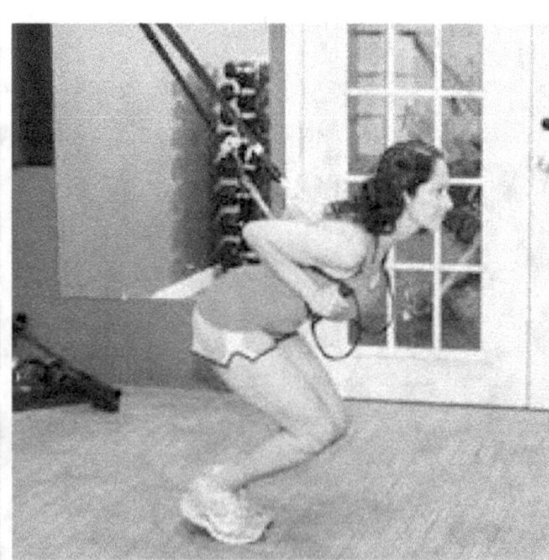

Sprinter Starts   Lower Body

This is one of my favorite movements because it improves strength, stability, and power, all with one movement. It's easy to modify and progress. It's also a fun exercise. It will help develop a strong leg extension that is required for forward propulsion, and pushing up hills.

Primary Focus: Legs and hips.
Setup: Straps fully extended.

1. Face away with the straps underneath your arms. Place the handles between your thumbs and index fingers, and with your elbows bent at your side, lean forward into the straps.
2. Go down into the movement by taking a large step back with one leg, allowing the front leg to bend.
3. Come back to the starting position by pushing back up through the front leg, and then finish the movement by driving the knee of what was the back leg up and toward your chest (like a person sprinting from the starting blocks).
4. Repeat all repetitions on one side, rest, and then switch legs.

The handles should be in your armpits. It's OK if your heels come off the ground when you're leaning forward, but your body should stay straight like a board. Start slowly and increase the speed of the movement when you feel comfortable. To progress this exercise further, add a hop.

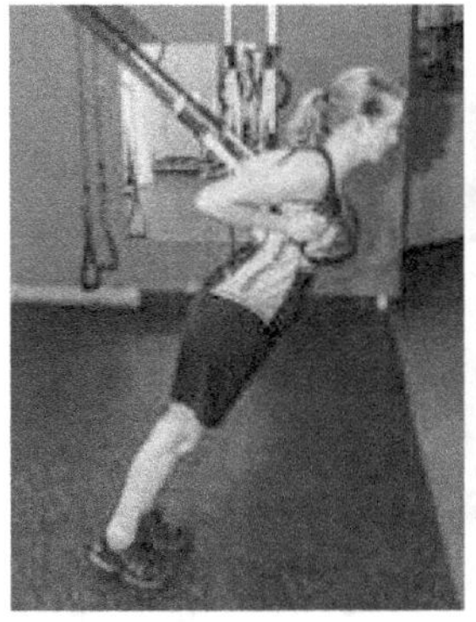 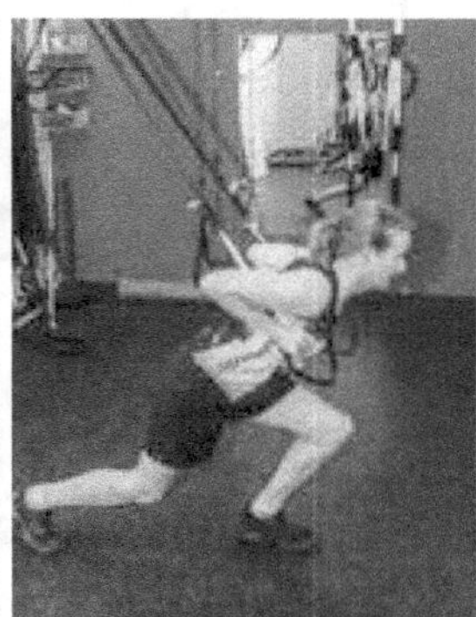 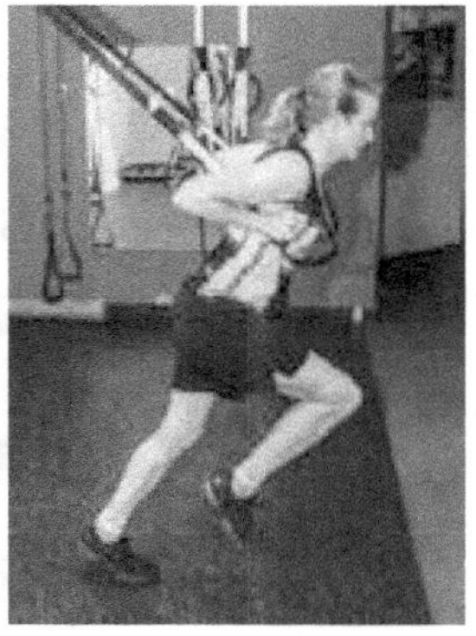

Suspended Reverse Lunge Lower Body

This is a reverse lunge with the foot of the non-working leg suspended in both cradles. This takes away the support of the ground at the bottom of the movement, and adds a degree of instability. This exercise will help both strengthen and stabilize the leg and hip muscles all the way from the feet to the hips. It will also be a balance challenge for most of you. Hold a dowel, bar, or hiking pole to help with balance if you need to, until you can master the balance through the whole movement.

Primary Focus: Legs and hips.
Setup: Straps fully extended and six inches off the ground.

1. Start by facing away from the anchor with the toes of one foot in both cradles of the suspended trainer.
2. Drop down into the movement by pushing back with the foot that is in the cradle, allowing the front leg to bend and your hips to drop down toward the floor.
3. Return to the starting position by stepping back up through the front leg, and bringing the back leg back in line with the front leg. Perform a set of consecutive repetitions on one side, then repeat on the other side.

The work is to be performed by the supporting leg. Minimize the weight you're putting on the strap of the suspended leg to the extent you are able. Make sure you have mastered the reverse lunge before progressing to the suspended variation.

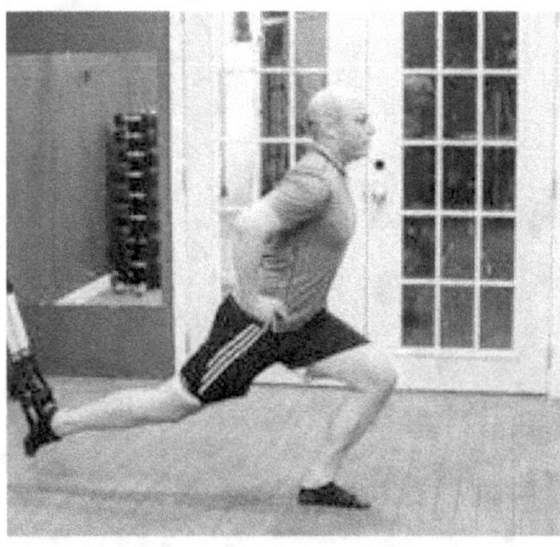
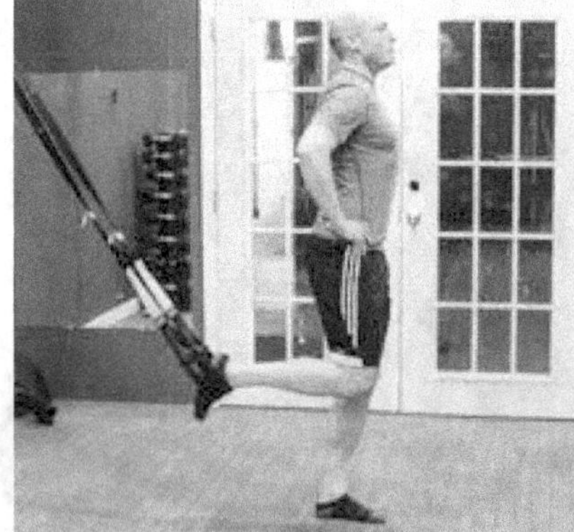

Suspended Power Lunge — Lower Body

An explosive movement that will increase strength and power of the hips and legs. The legs and hips must stay aligned while absorbing impact, decelerating body mass, and then producing explosive power to push the body back up—all with just one leg. The impact and high force generated are great for bone health.

Primary Focus: Legs and Hips.
Setup: Straps fully extended and six inches off the ground.

1. Face away from the anchor on one leg, with the foot of the other leg suspended in both cradles.
2. Drop down into the movement by pushing back with the foot that's in the cradle, allowing the front leg to bend and your hips to drop down toward the floor.
3. Now, when you get to the bottom, power back up with as much acceleration as you can produce. Push through the front leg as you pull the suspended knee back in line with the supporting knee. The result should be a hop or jump off the ground.

Explode on the way up. Make sure to control the landing, and maintain good form on the way back down. Knee stays over the foot, and your torso stays straight up and down.

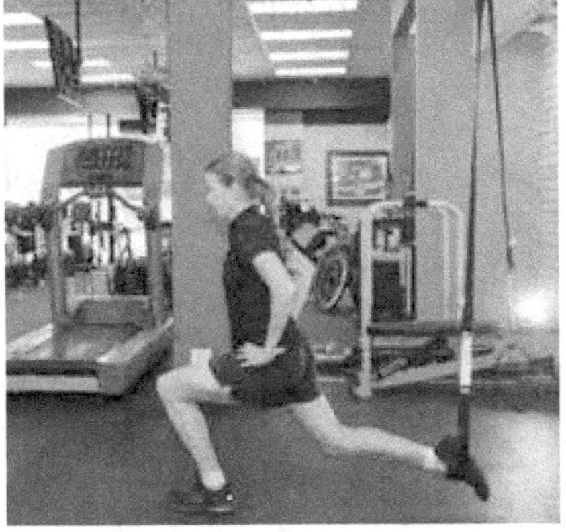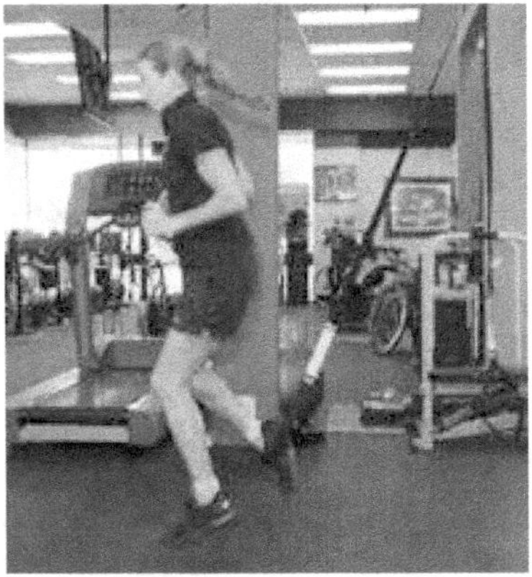

Master the suspended lunge movement before attempting the suspended power lunge.

Single-Leg Squat
Lower Body

You may have heard of the pistol squat. This is a version of it. You will need optimal strength and stability to descend into the lowest version of this movement. The good news is that using the straps will help you maintain form as you progress and increase the depth you can descend to.

Primary Focus: Legs and Hips.
Setup: Straps mid-length.

1. Facing the anchor point, keep the arms relaxed and shoulders back, lift up one leg, and support your body weight with your other leg.
2. Descend toward the floor with only the supporting leg. Keep an upright torso and good posture. Use the straps for balance, but don't lean back on them too much. Use your legs.
3. At the bottom, push yourself back up through the supporting leg, exhaling as you rise. Make sure you keep your shoulders back, core engaged, and head in line with the spine and torso (don't look down during the movement)

If you are having trouble with this one start by focusing on controlling the descent and holding the endzone at the bottom for several seconds, instead of doing the full movement. This helps develop the mobility and motor pattern to progress to the full movement.

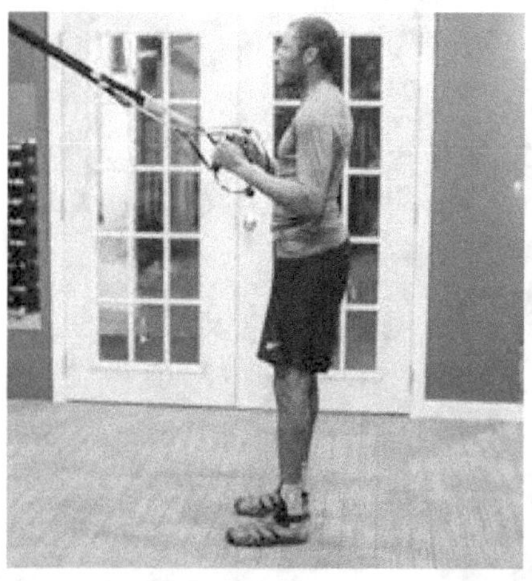 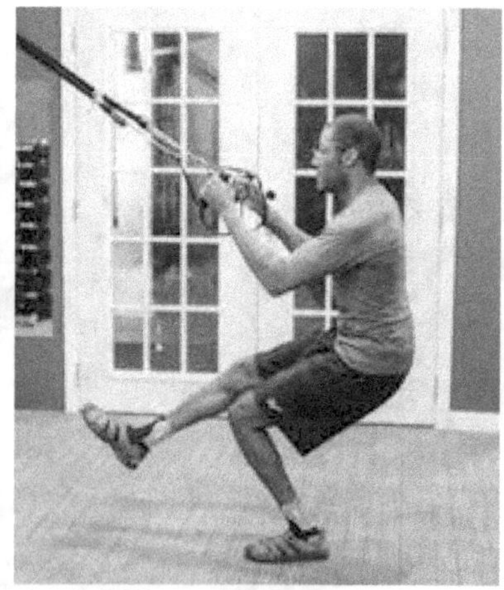

Split Squat Jump

This movement is great for hip and leg strength and works the hips and legs in an opposing movement pattern which is relevant high intensity(especially out of the saddle) efforts. It will help develop power in the legs and hips, and help improve and maintain bone density as well.

Primary Focus: Legs and hips.
Setup: Straps fully extended.

1. Face the anchor, hold the straps, and assume a long split-stride position, with one leg forward and one behind you.
2. Keep the arms relaxed and shoulders back, and drop the back knee down to the floor.
3. When you reach the bottom, immediately power back up through the hips and legs, jump as high as you are able, and quickly switch legs while you're in the air. When you land, the leg that was behind you is now in front, and vice versa.

Your jump should be straight up, and you should land in the same spot with the legs reversed. Keep your knees in line with your feet and your weight over your legs and feet.

**Make sure you've mastered proper technique of the split-stance squat before adding the jump to*

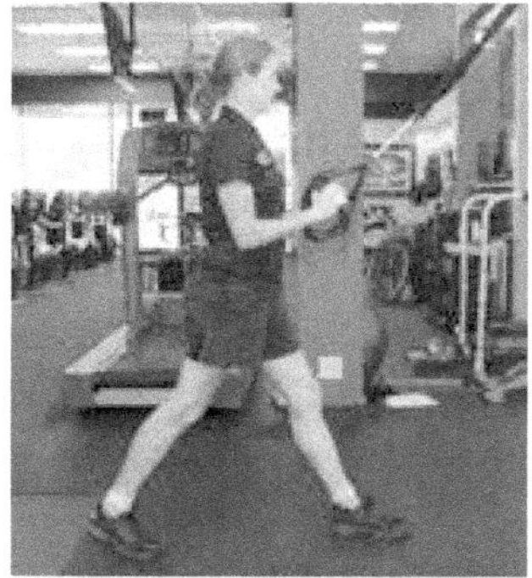
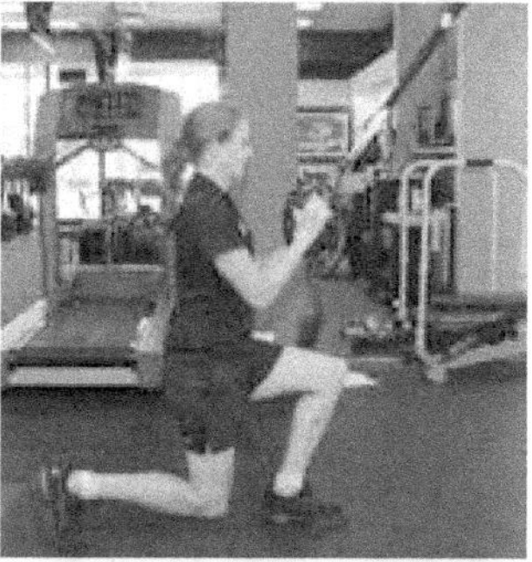
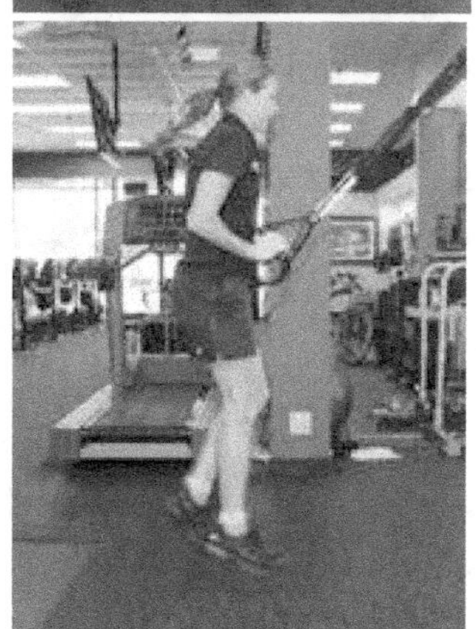
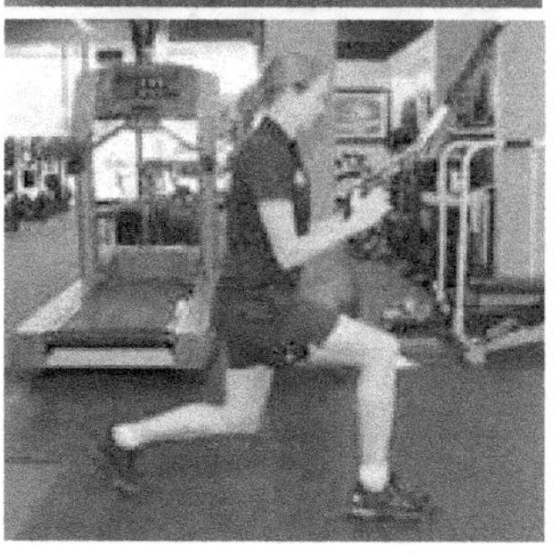

Skaters

Lower Body

This movement develops leg and hip strength and power. It also develops stability, and the ability to control and decelerate your body weight while keeping your ankle, knee, and hip aligned. It's a fun movement where you can catch some air and increase the distance you jump from side to side as you get stronger.

Primary Focus: Legs and hips.
Setup: Straps fully extended.

1. Face the anchor, holding the straps. Step out to the side with one leg, and drop down into a lateral lunge movement.
2. Power back up through that leg, pushing yourself over and landing on the opposite leg. As you descend on the supporting leg, cross the unsupported leg behind you.
3. Push back up through the supporting leg and repeat. Make sure your knee stays right over and in line with your foot as you are controlling your deceleration and then pushing off.

As you get proficient with this one, increase the distance you step out to the side. To make it even harder, add a jump to it. Spring yourself up from the side to catch some air in the middle before landing on the other side.

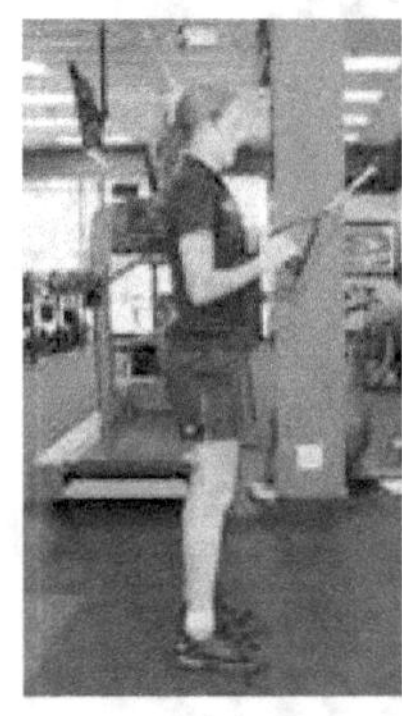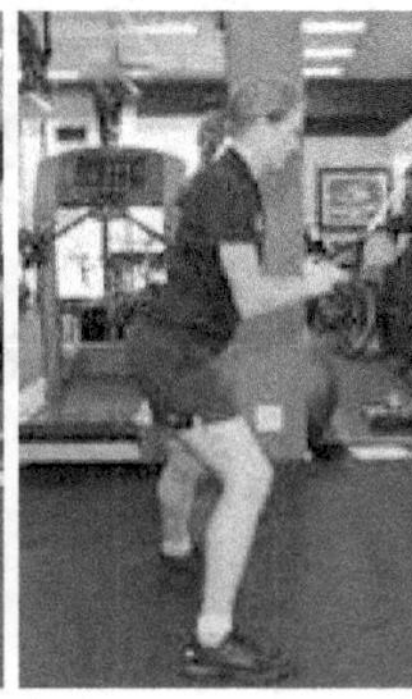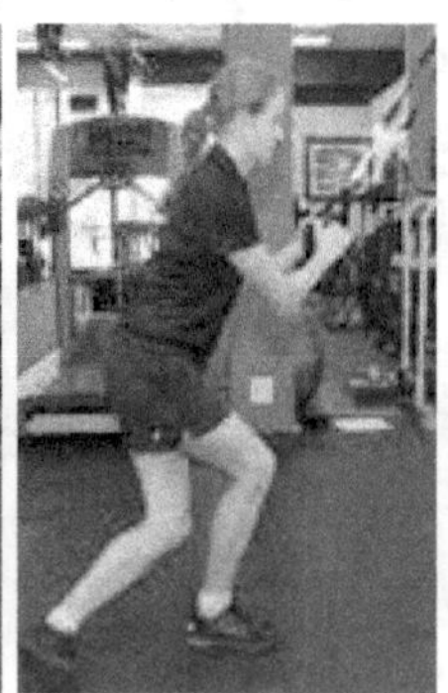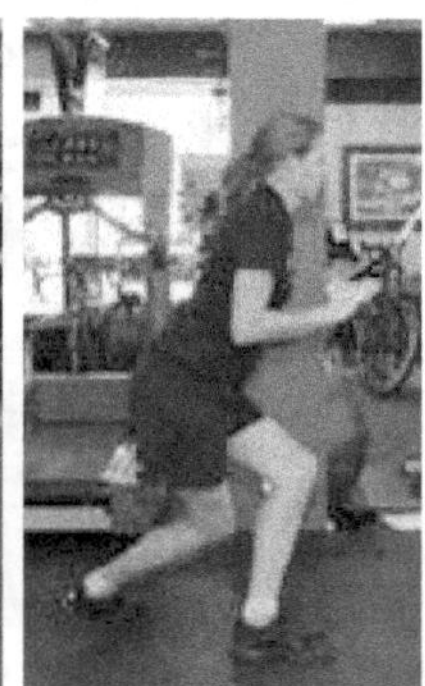

Master the crossover lunge before doing skaters.

Jump Squat

Lower Body

This exercise will develop explosive power of the hips and legs. It will train your muscles to be able to fire more of the larger muscle fibers more quickly. The impact is good for your bones, and catching air is fun!

Focus: Legs and hips.
Setup: Straps fully extended.

1. Facing the anchor, hold the straps, and stand with your feet a little wider than shoulder width.
2. Keep the arms relaxed and shoulders back, and squat down toward the floor.
3. When you reach the bottom, immediately power back up through the hips and legs, and jump as high as you are able. Keep your weight over your feet when going into and coming out of the squat. Your knees should be directly over your feet, not out in front of them

Give this movement some zip by jumping side to side, or pulling your knees up toward your chest when you are airborne.
This movement can be also be progressed by doing it freestanding, holding weight, or wearing a weight vest.

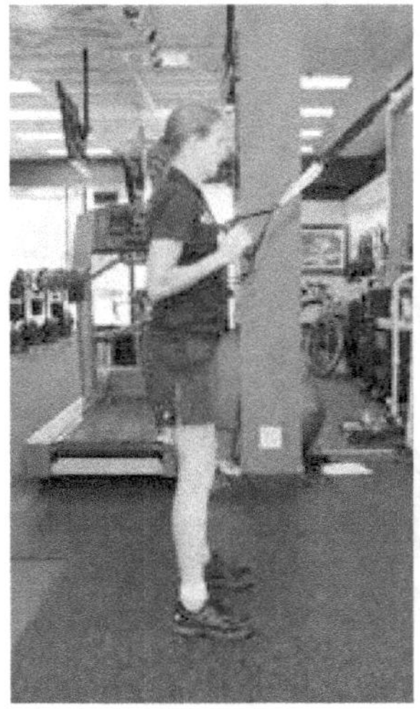
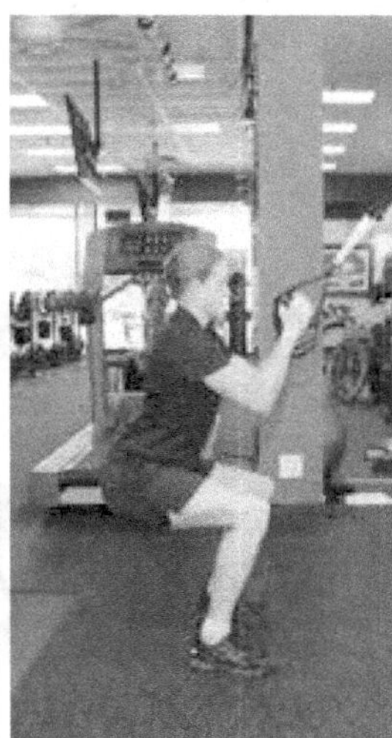
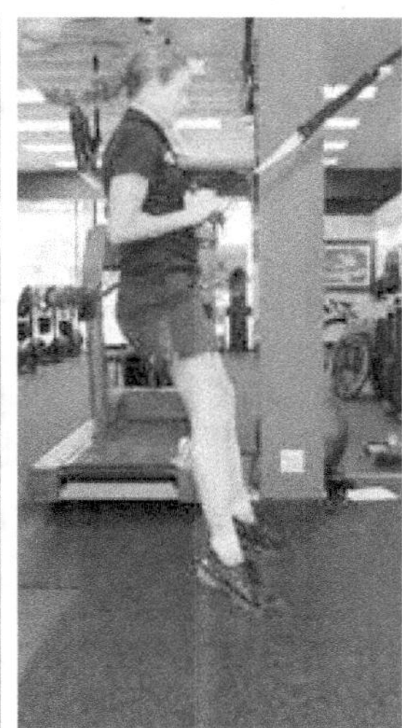

Overhead Squat

Lower Body

This is a challenging movement that requires optimum strength, stability, and mobility throughout the ankles, hips, torso, and shoulders. This movement develops and maintains a strong and solid movement foundation that will support all demands of strength and endurance training and activity

Focus: Legs, hips, upper torso, arms
Setup: Straps fully extended.

1. Facing the anchor, with a shoulder-width stance. Place your hands in the straps with your fingers extended, the backs of your hands pressing into the foot cradles, and arms extended straight above your head.
2. Drop your hips down into your squat while keeping your arms extended straight above your head, applying light pressure on the straps with the back of your hands. Descend below parallel if able to do so while maintaining form.
3. Immediately stand back up by pushing though the legs and hips while maintaining the arms overhead.

Keep your torso vertical and knees and hands directly over your feet during the squat. Your arms should not come forward, and your knees should not extend in front of your toes.

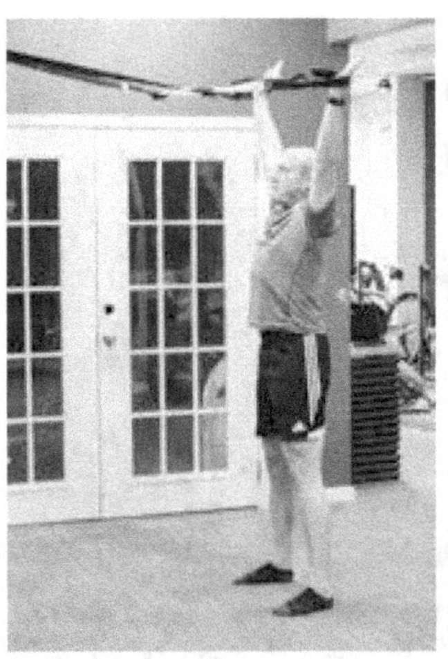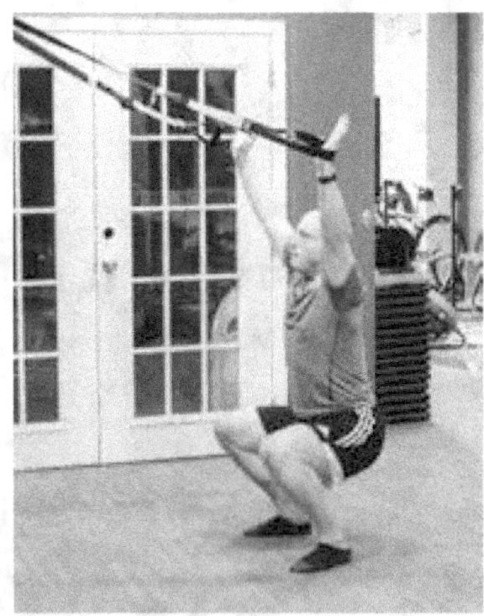

Plank
Core

This is a great all-purpose movement, as a strong core is beneficial to general strength for all activities as well as for good posture. For cycling performance, it will build the strength to stabilize and create a solid center of mass to drive movement. This
includes maintenance of form during fatigue, and power transfer
through the core during hard efforts, hills or adverse terrain.

Focus: Core, Arms and Shoulders

1. Start in a ground position facing down.
2. Consciously contract all the muscles you can feel, from your
   toes to your shoulders.
3. Raise your body up as one unit, so you are contacting the
   ground with only your forearms and toes.
4. Make sure your body forms a straight line from your shoulders to your ankles.
5. Engage your core by sucking your belly button to your spine.
6. Hold with good form until you get tired

Ground Based Variations- *Modified, Standard, Straight Arm
and Side Plank.*

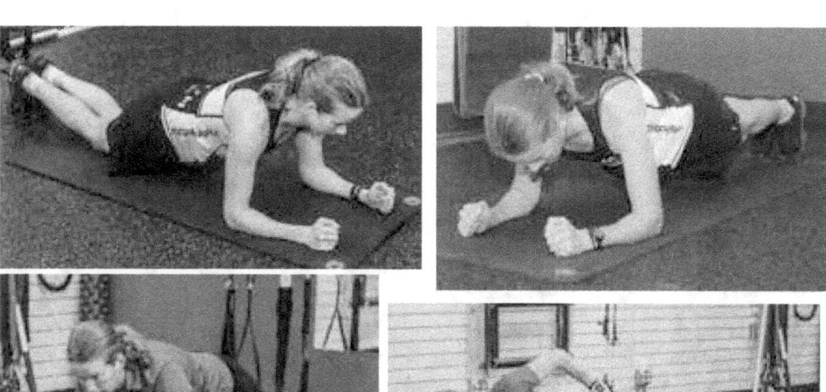

Bicycle Kicks   Core

The hip-flexion movement (when the knee is pulled toward the chest) targets the core and hip flexors. Strengthening these can improve your ability to drive you knee up and forward. This can benefit activities such as throwing a leg over the bike, clearing obstacles on or off the bike, and even adding power to the up-swing in your pedal stroke.

Focus: Core and Hip Flexors
Setup: Straps fully extended and six inches off the ground.

1. Lie on your back with your feet in the cradles and your knees slightly bent.
2. Before you start the movement, make sure you engage your core (think about tightening your stomach muscles as if someone was going to poke you in the stomach).
3. Alternate pulling each knee toward your chest as you extend the opposite leg.

The suspended bicycle kick is a great exercise for a beginner, and will help you learn to engage your hip flexors, which will result in better running mechanics. You don't need a suspended trainer to do this one, but having one helps the beginner master the movement by

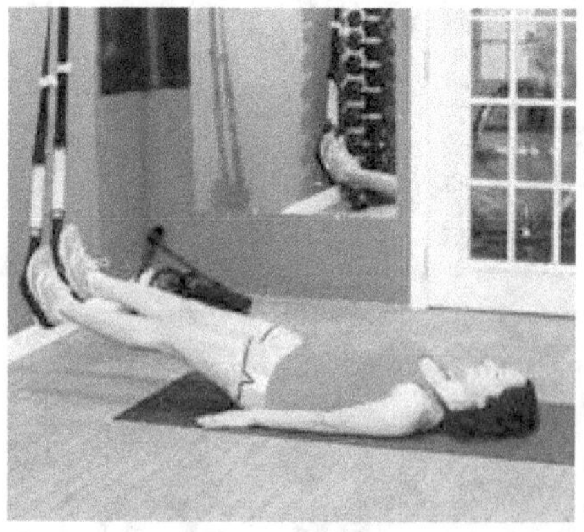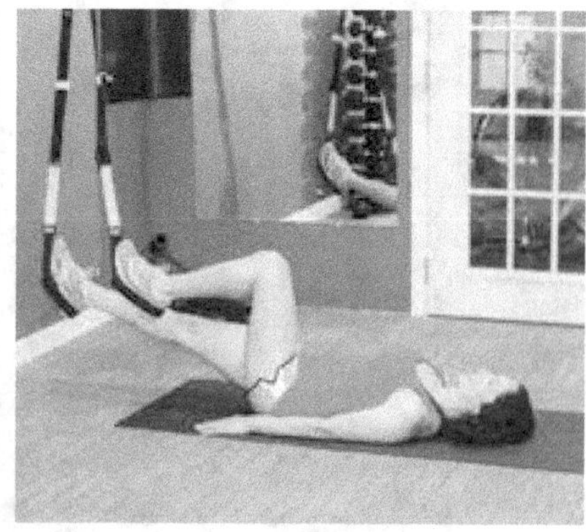

assisting with supporting some of the weight of the legs.

Suspended Hip Raise Core

Develops a solid foundation through the back side of the core, which includes your torso and hips.

Focus: Hamstrings and hips.
Setup: Straps fully extended and six inches off the ground.

1. Lie on your back with your feet in the cradles and your knees slightly bent. Your arms should be extended and at your sides on the mat.
2. Push your heels into the cradles to lift your hips off the floor. Focus on relaxed arms and pushing through the hips and heels.
3. Descend back down, keeping a stable position with your upper torso.

Progress by adding more knee bend to your starting position, which will let you push your hips higher off the ground.

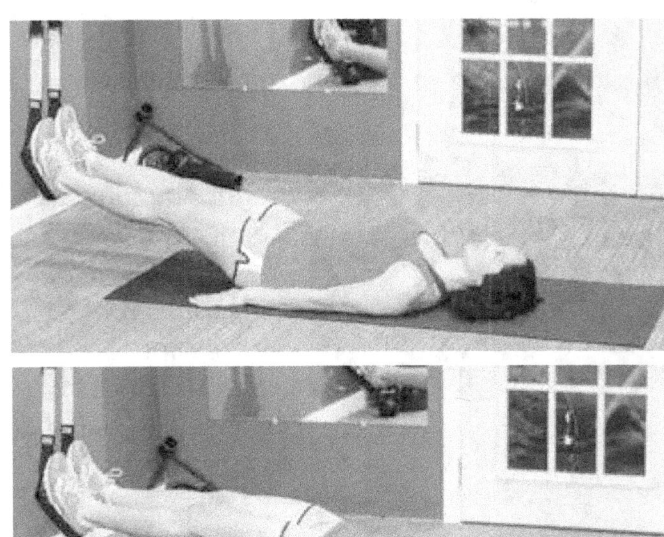

Lateral Hip Raise
Core

This is an excellent movement to strengthen hip stabilizers, which are important for strong hip and gait mechanics during walking and running. This may not transfer directly to the up and down motion of the pedal stroke. However, highly specialized cyclists in particular, may need have weakness in this area and this movement could benefit overall movement and gait mechanics.

Focus: Core and Obliques and Gluts

1. Get on your side, supporting yourself through your forearm by placing the elbow directly below your shoulder. The bottom knee should be bent and inline with your elbow, and the upper leg should be straight.
2. Push your hips off the ground through your downed knee, and simultaneously lift your top leg while keeping it straight.
3. Descend back down and repeat for the targeted amount of repetitions or time.

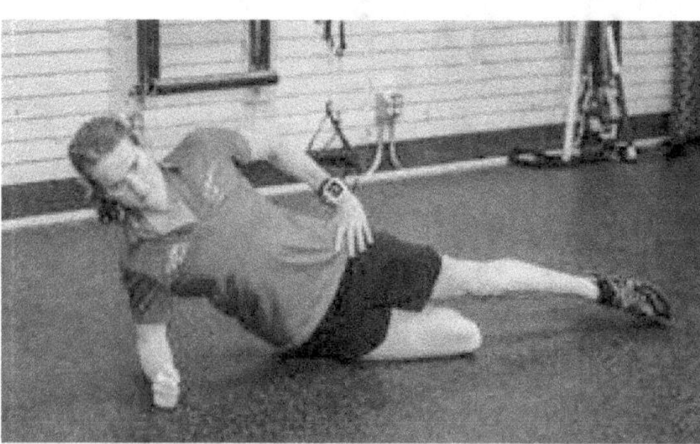

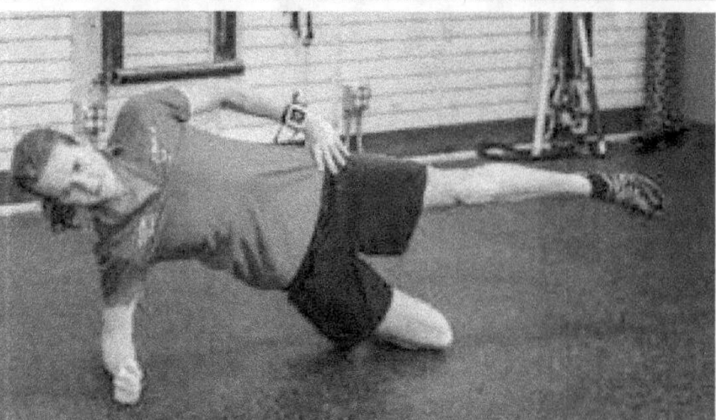

This movement can be surprisingly challenging if you're doing it right. You can make it easier by allowing your top leg and foot to maintain contact with the floor. You can assist the hip lift by also pressing with that foot into the floor.

Half Get-Up Core

This is a fundamental movement that I include with some progression in almost all my programs. This is the level 1 progression, and the best one with which to start. Everyone should have the ability to easily and properly get up off the floor from a position of lying down, and this move will develop both the strength and motor patterns to do so. It will also develop a solid foundation to build on when progressing to more advanced variations.

Focus: Core

1. Lie on your back with one leg straight and the other bent. The arm on the bent-leg side should point straight up to the ceiling.
2. Start by lifting your shoulders off the ground as if you were doing a crunch, and continue ascending by pushing through the downed elbow. Keep your straight arm vertical and pointing at the ceiling the entire time. Lift your chest and squeeze your shoulder blades together at the top.
3. Perform the desired amount of repetitions on one side. Rest, and then switch sides.

To make it harder, hold a weight in the hand that is reaching up. Keep it light; you don't need much. A light dumbbell, kettlebell, or even a can of soup will work. If you build to more than ten repetitions, move on to the next advanced progression.

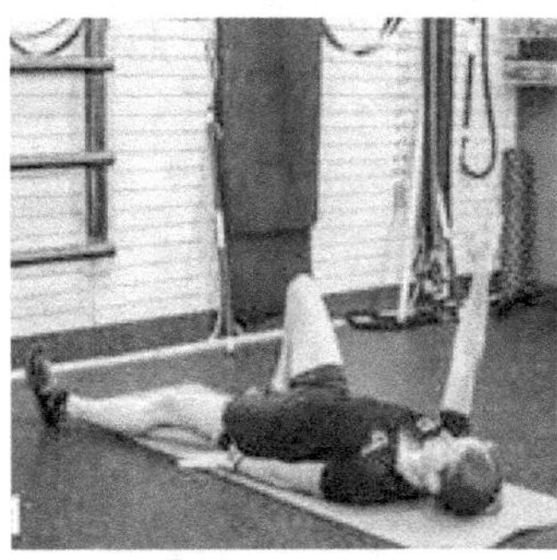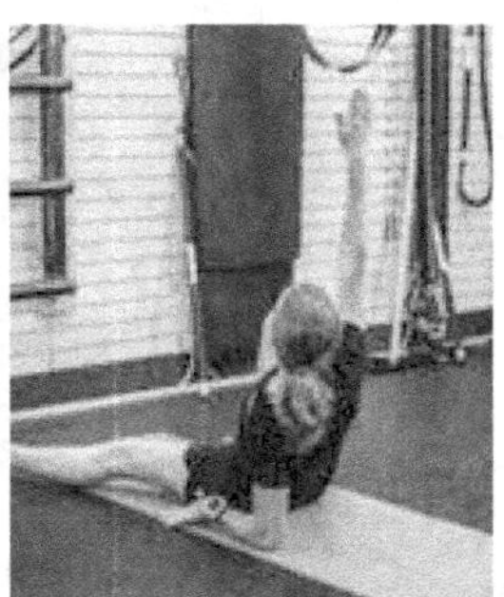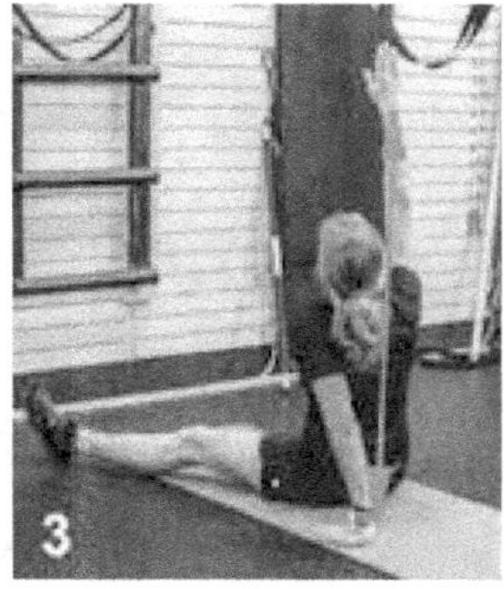

Half-Kneeling Rollout   Core

The core is what drives the arm movement in this exercise. Power is transferred through the core between the arms and hips, which are fixed to the floor. This movement is a good complement to movements such as the crunch and sit up(next page), which also work the core, but tend to isolate the ab muscles more.

Focus: Core
Setup: Straps fully extended.

1. Get on one knee and hold the straps in front of you. You will be supporting your weight on the downed knee and have the other leg right in front of you with the foot on the floor (you may use a folded- up towel, mat, or pad under the downed knee for comfort).
2. Now push the straps away from you, and extend the torso and arms out in front and slightly to the side.
3. Return to the starting position by pulling yourself back up-right through your core. Do this by tightening your stomach muscles to drive the movement though the core and torso.
4. Do a full set on one side. Switch sides and do a full set on the other side.

Before you start the movement, make sure the muscles of the supporting hip are tight, and the hip is inline with your knee and torso. Squeeze the muscles in your butt to

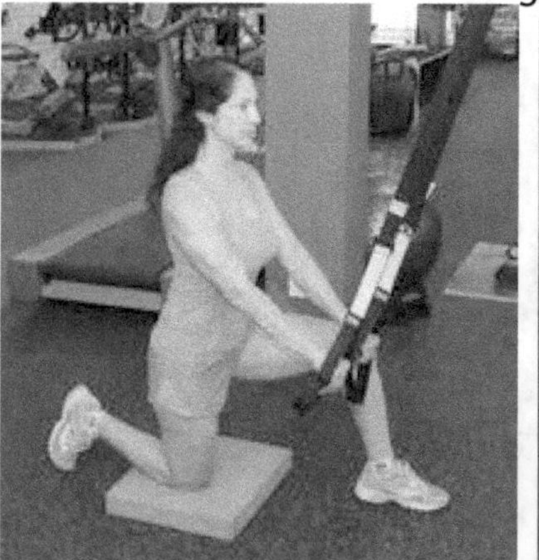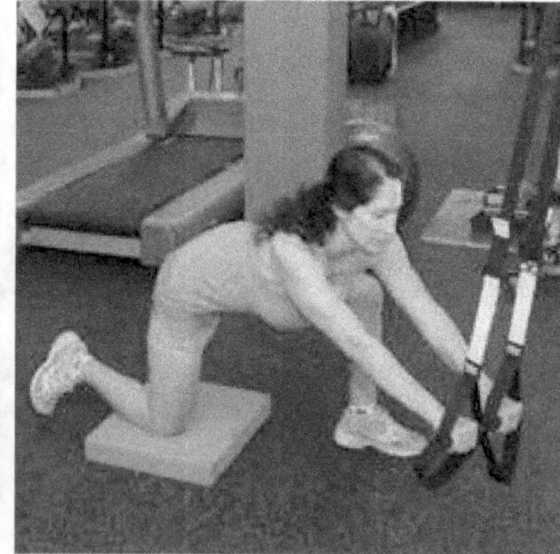

Crunch and Suspended Sit-Up Core

Develops all-around core and hip-flexor strength. This will give you a solid foundation that can better support the demands of all activities.

Primary Focus: Core, Hip flexors to assist the sit-up movement.
Setup: Straps fully extended and six inches off the ground.

Crunch:

1. Lie on your back with your heels in the cradles, arms extended, and reach toward the ceiling.
2. Keep your arms vertical, and reach straight up toward the celling until your shoulder blades are off the ground.
3. Come back down, and as soon as you feel the floor with your upper back again, crunch back up to the top. This is a small but effective range of motion.

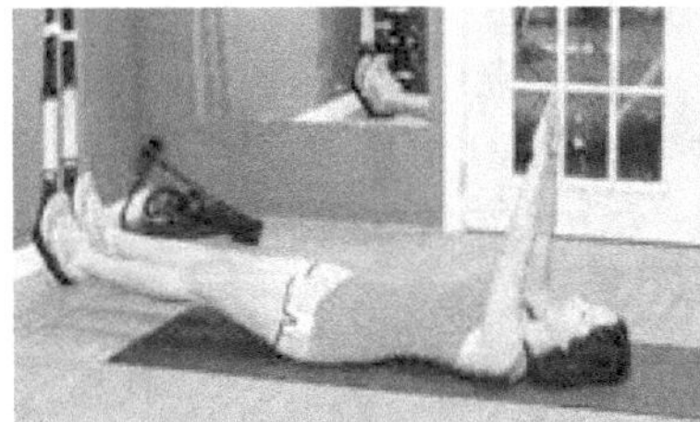 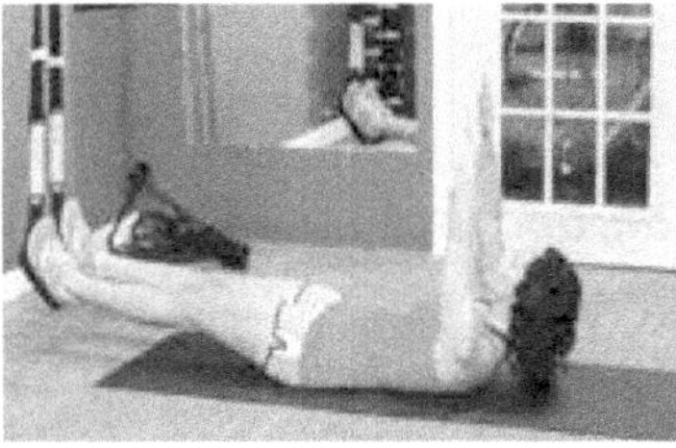

Sit-Up:

Instead of stopping to come back down when you feel your shoulder blades are no longer touching the floor, continue to ascend until your torso is vertical, keeping the arms extended upward toward the ceiling.

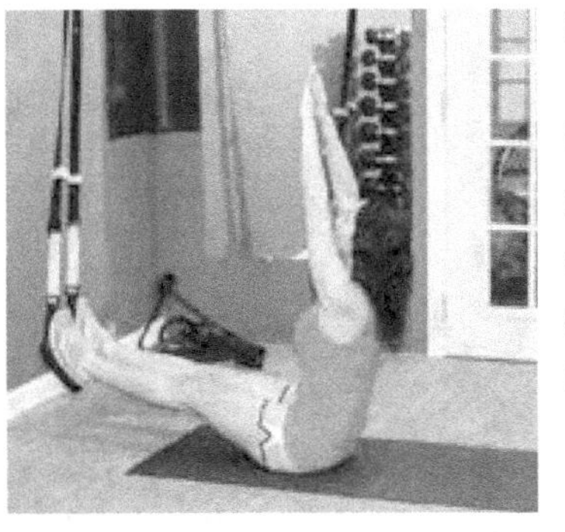

When doing the sit-up, strive to obtain full extension and reach for the ceiling at the top. That little extra move will do wonders in developing muscles that will support good posture.

Suspended Plank Core

This is a step up from the ground bases variations. If you're new to the plank exercise, start with the variations on the previous page instead of in the straps. Progress to the straps after you feel you've mastered the traditional version of the plank.

Focus: Core, Arms and Shoulders.
Setup: Straps fully extended and six inches off the ground.

1. Get on your hands and knees, facing forward and down so that your head is in alignment with your neck and spine, with your toes in the cradles.
2. Preload the core by tightening the muscles in your mid-section, and straighten your legs to lift your knees off the ground. Your body should be straight like a table. Your elbows should be directly underneath your shoulders, and your head inline with your spine.
3. Time yourself, and hold until you feel fatigued.

This exercise is all about form! Hips need to stay up, don't let the lower back sag, and keep shoulders soft and back flat (no rounding the back). Doing this one in front of a mirror will allow you to self- monitor your form. If you feel you can't hold your form, stop immediately and mark that as your time.

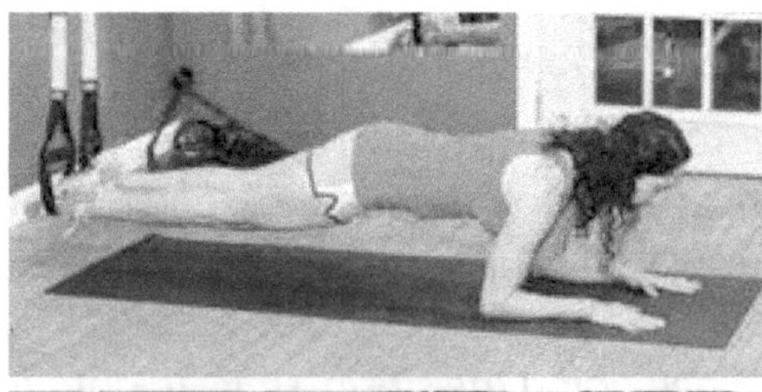

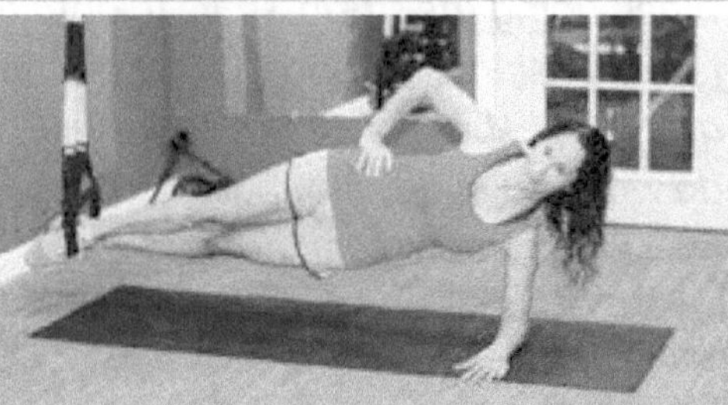

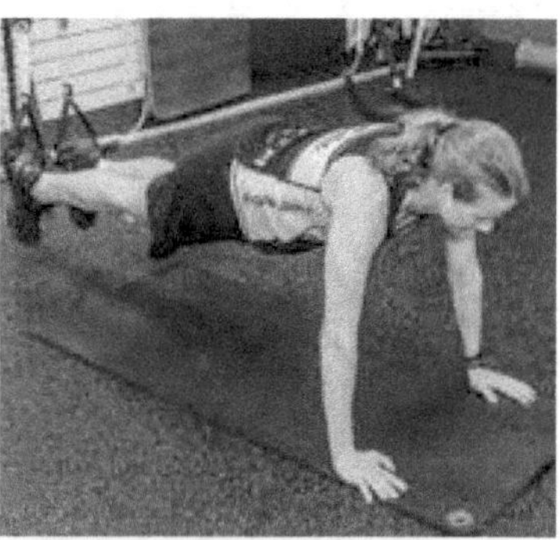

Suspended Variations - *Standard, Side and Straight Arm*

Mountain Climbers

Core

You are basically adding a leg movement to a straight-arm plank. It's
actually more of a movement but
also helps to develop power transfer
through the core. Whith this one
the hands are fixed, and the legs
performing the movement.

Focus: Core, Hip Flexors and Arms

1. Get into a straight-arm plank
   position.
2. Maintain your body position to
   be straight like a surfboard and
   alternate pulling your knees toward your chest, one at a time.
3. Repeat for targeted repetitions
   or time. Keep your butt down
   and body straight! A common
   thing I see is that when people
   get tired they end up lifting
   their hips higher because it
   makes it easier. Don't do it.

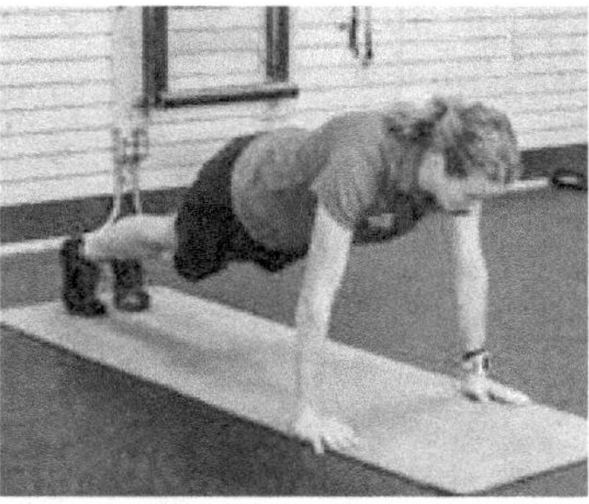
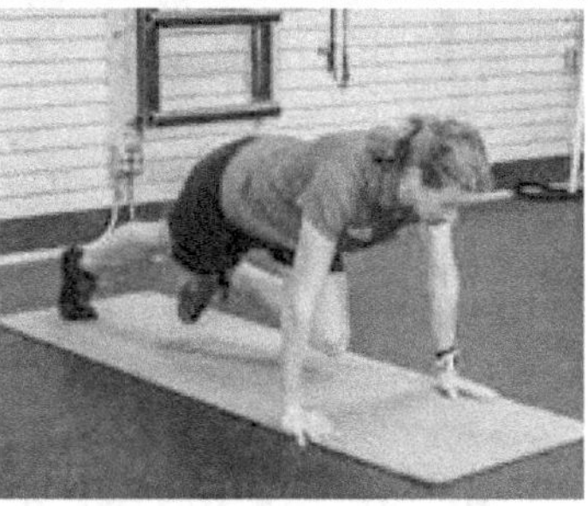
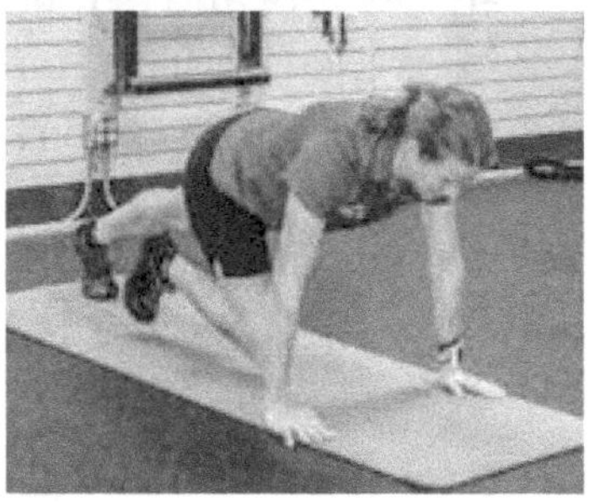

*To make it harder, increase the speed until you are simultaneously
bringing one leg forward and the other back. Your feet will touch the
ground on both ends of the range of motion on this version.*

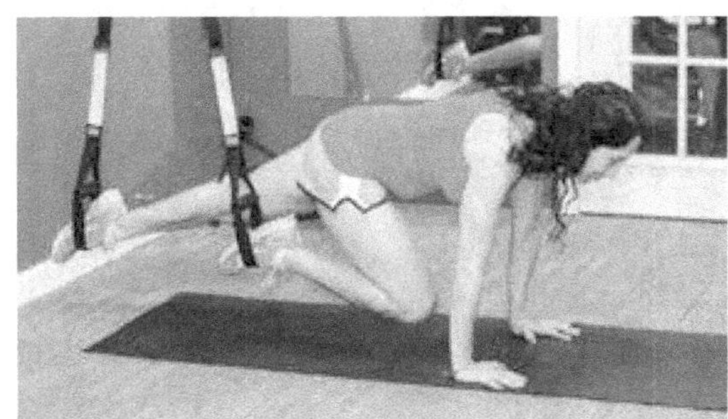

*There are also two
progressions using the
suspended trainer: one
with your hands sus-
pended, and one with
your feet suspended.*

Tall Kneeling Rollout

Core

This is a more advanced version of the half-kneeling rollout. The core drives the arm movement in both cases, but this version requires more strength because you don't have a foot forward to help support the resistance, as you extend out during the movement. Being able to hold your position with an extended body helps develop a strong and stable core and upper body.

Focus: Core, Arms and Back
Setup: Straps fully extended.

1. Face the suspended trainer, kneeling on both knees, torso upright, and holding the straps (place a pad, mat, or rolled-up towel under the knees for comfort).
2. Maintain good posture by making yourself tall, keeping shoulders relaxed, chest out, and looking forward. Tighten the core, lean forward, and extend the arms out in front of you.
3. Return to the start by pulling up with both your hips and core and bringing the arms back toward the body.

It will get hard quickly as your body gets longer. Extend out to a position you can maintain with good form. If you feel any pain in your lower back, don't go out as far, or skip this one.

Starting farther out will be harder, and starting farther underneath the anchor point will be easier (refer to chapter 3).

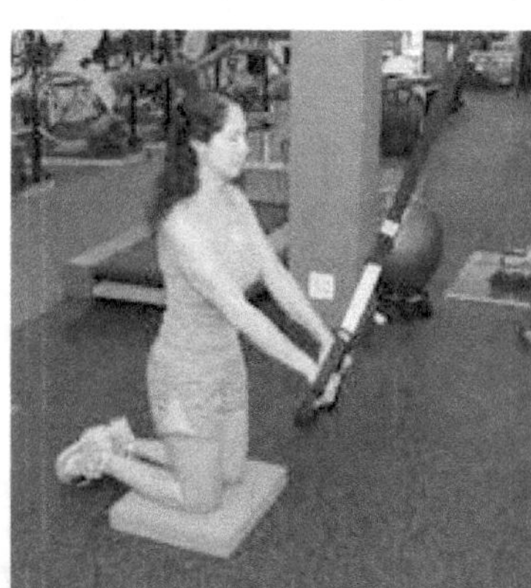
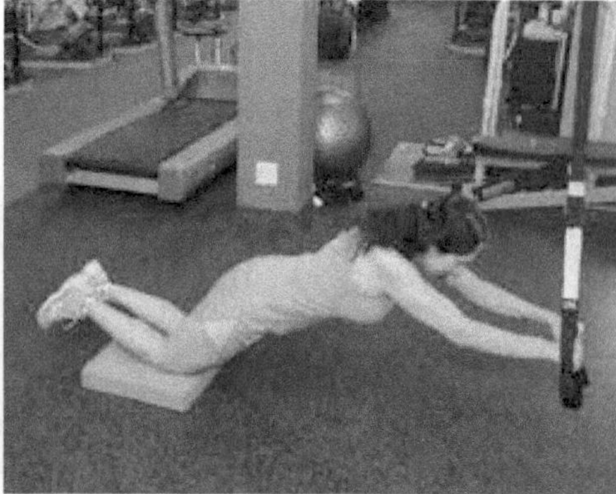

Atomic Crunches Core

Trains the hip flexors and deep core muscles to work together in a strong, powerful movement. This movement will help develop power transfer through the core. It will also develop hip flexor strength, which will strengthen the drive (when you pull the knee back through), which is especially relevant in sprinting or hard climbing efforts.

Primary Focus: Core and hip flexors, Arms
Setup: Straps fully extended and six inches off the ground.

1. Face away from the suspended trainer on your hands and knees, with your toes in the cradles, right underneath the anchor. Your hands should be directly underneath your shoulders.
2. To start, straighten your legs, which is going to lift your knees off the ground. Keep a slight bend in the elbows, push the hips upward, and pull the knees toward the chest.
3. Finish with both knees bent and close to your chest, arms slightly bent and directly underneath your shoulders.
4. Extend the legs backward to return to the starting position. Keep your core tight, and don't let your back or hips sag during this exercise.

For some extra bang, alternate repetitions with the suspended floor push-up. For example, instead of 15 repetitions of atomic crunches, alternate between the two movements and perform 8 of each.

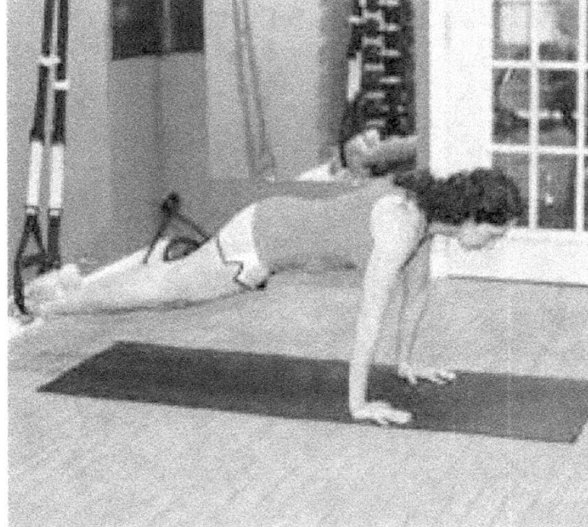 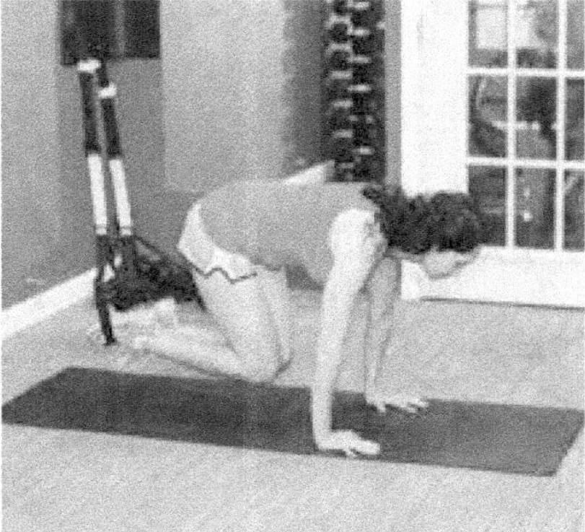

Suspended Pike

Core

This is a challenging movement that will develop your overall dynamic core strength, as well as your ability to support and stabilize your body weight with your upper body while the lower body moves. This will translate into a solid foundation that will support all your activities and endeavors.

Primary Focus: Core and Hip Flexors, Arms
Setup: Straps fully extended and six inches off the ground.

1. Face away from the suspended trainer on your hands and knees, with your toes in the cradles, right underneath the anchor. Your hands should be slightly wider than shoulder width, and your thumbs should be aligned with your chest.
2. To get in starting position, simply straighten your legs, which is going to lift your knees off the ground.
3. Pull your legs toward your chest by driving your hips upward toward the ceiling.
4. At the top of the movement, pause and slowly go back down to the starting position. Keep your core tight, and don't let your back or hips sag during this exercise. Your hands should remain in line with your shoulders, and the line between them, would be directly under your chest (not your face).

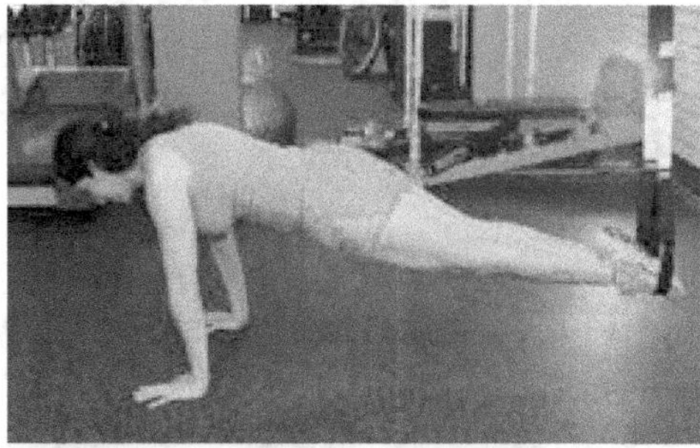

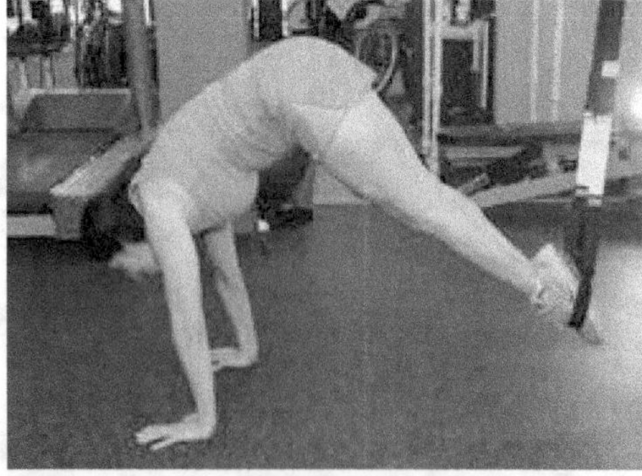

Starting farther out will be harder, and starting farther underneath the anchor point will be easier (refer to chapter 3).

Squat Press
Whole Body

This is a great full-body exercise that will challenge those at a beginner-to-intermediate level. It can also serve as a functional warm-up, or part of a circuit program for more advanced levels. It will provide some dynamic flexibility for those with tight shoulders and chest muscles.

Focus: Legs and Shoulders.
Setup: Straps fully extended.

1. Face away from the anchor with a handle in each hand and the straps on the outside of your arms and a slight forward lean. Start the movement by dropping your hips toward the floor.
2. At the lowest part of the movement, you should be on the balls of your feet and have a slight forward lean, elbows bent, and the handles in line with your shoulders. Push back up with your legs and hips, exhaling and pressing your arms overhead.
3. Your finishing position should be full extension of both your arms and legs, leaning slightly forward.

Try hard to obtain the full extension at the top of the movement. Think about squeezing your arms to your ears and reaching toward the sky.

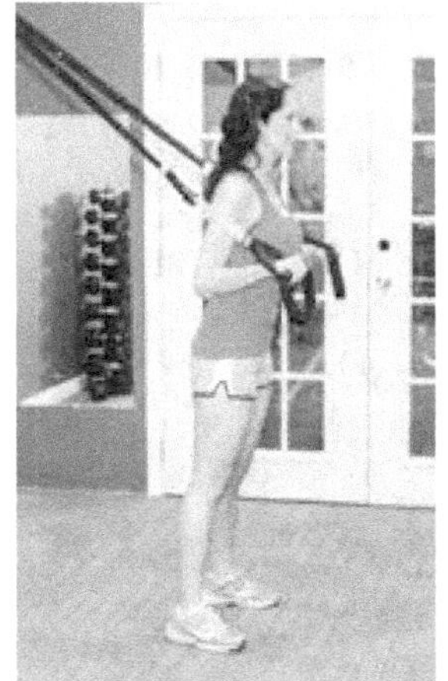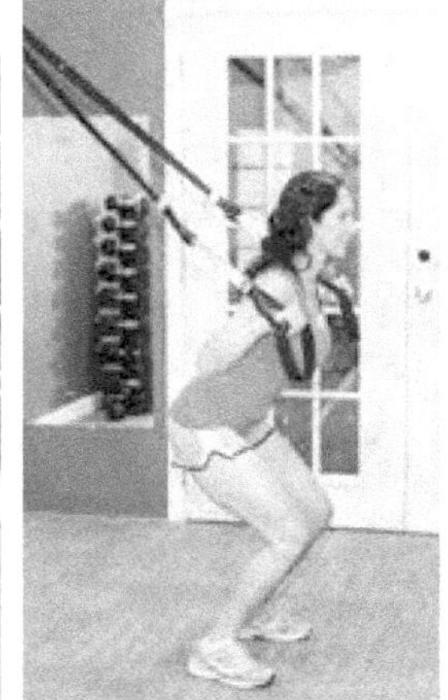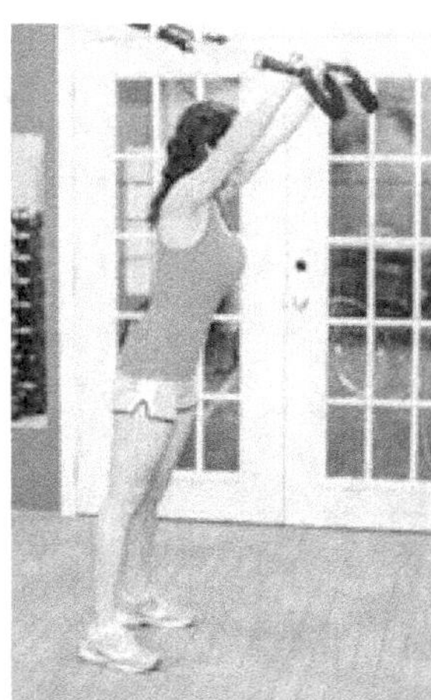

Squat Row Whole Body

This is an all-purpose foundational movement that reinforces squat form, while also targeting the chain of muscles in the back and torso that are responsible for good posture. This exercise will challenge those at a beginner-to-intermediate level, and can serve as a functional warm-up or part of a circuit program for more advanced levels

Focus: Legs and Back.
Setup: Straps fully extended.

1. Facing the anchor, hold the straps with a shoulder-width stance. Lean back slightly.
2. Sit down into the squat by dropping your hips down toward the floor. When you get to the bottom, your arms should be straight and extended in front of you.
3. Push yourself back up with your legs while simultaneously pulling your upper body toward the straps. Your finish position should be standing tall with elbows bent at your side.

Those who spend a lot of time at a desk or behind the wheel would benefit from combining the squat press on the previous page, which will help open up the chest and shoulders, with the squat row, which targets the large and small posture muscles.

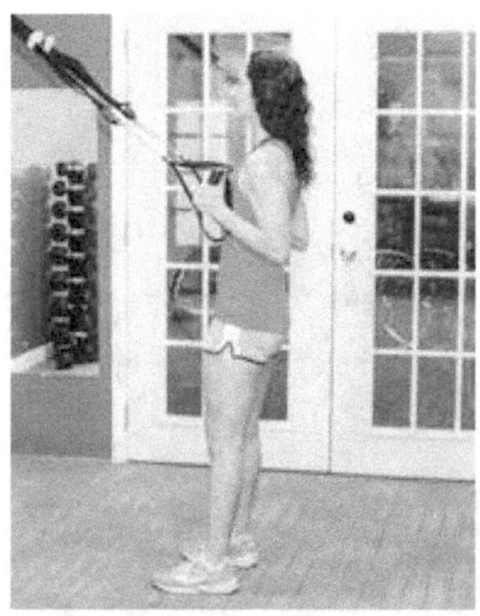 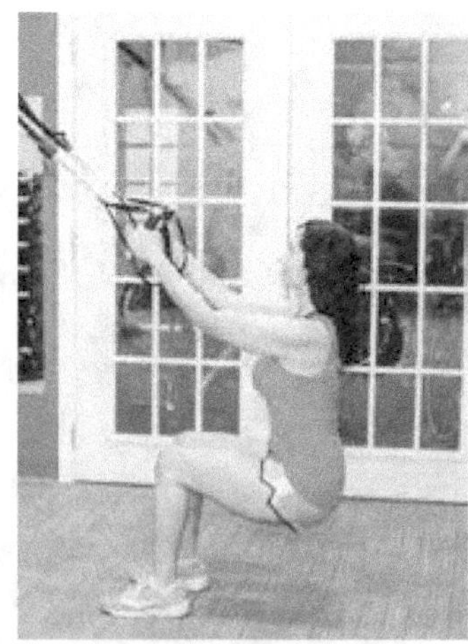

Squat to Reverse Fly   Whole Body

These two movements performed together will result in working many muscle groups at the same time. The reverse fly movement will help your posture, and adding the squat at the same time will get the entire chain of muscles in your back and torso working together.

Focus: Rear shoulders and legs.
Setup: Straps fully extended.

1. Facing the anchor, with a slightly wider than shoulder-width stance, hold the straps with your arms extended in front of you.
2. While keeping your arms straight, sit down into the squat. Go down as low as you feel comfortable with.
3. At the bottom, push back up, and when you get close to the top of the movement, immediately move your arms out to the side until they are in line with your shoulders.

Get into an amount of lean that will load the desired amount of weight onto the reserve fly movement. You will still be leaning back to some extent during the squat, but that's OK. Also, keep the movement controlled, and don't use momentum to swing you back up from the squat. Make your legs and hips do the work.

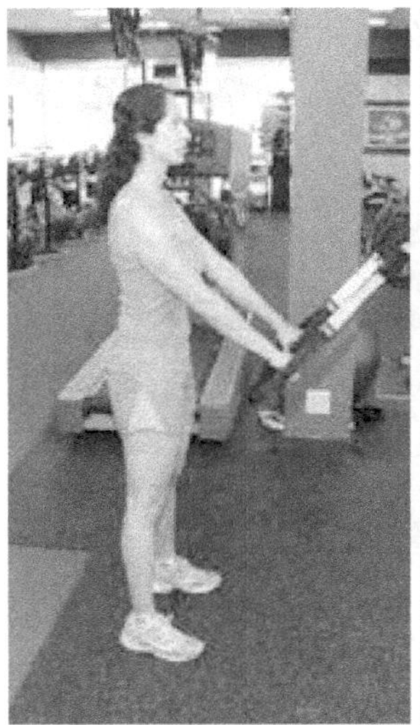
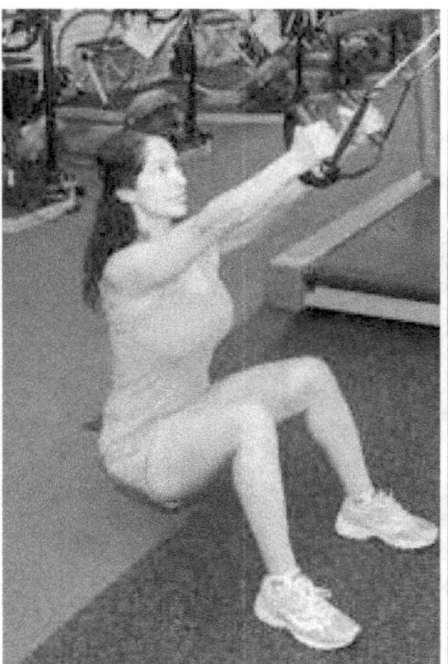
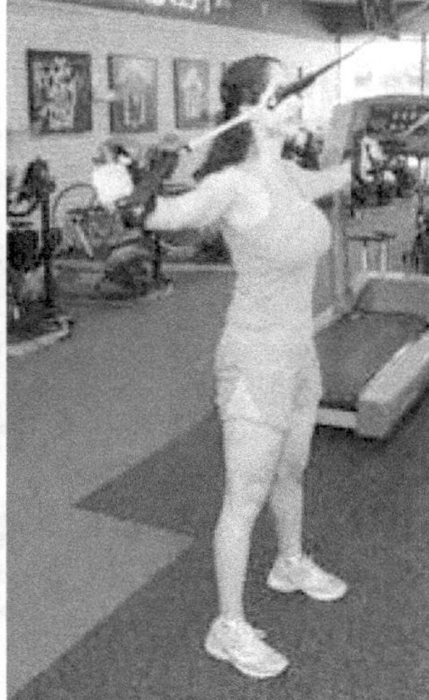

Suspended Get-Up Whole Body

This is a great all-purpose, foundational movement combines a single-leg squat, row, and triceps extension movement all in one. This is an excellent full-body movement that requires aspects of stability, strength, and mobility.

Focus: Legs, back, and arms.
Setup: Straps fully extended.

1. Sit on the floor facing in and holding the straps. The straps should have tension on them at this point. Extend one leg straight in front of you with the other leg bent at the knee.
2. Start the movement by pushing through the hip of the bent leg while simultaneously pulling yourself with your arms. Keep good posture (shoulders back, head looking forward) while making the ascent.
3. When you reach the top, your feet will be together. Immediately continue into a triceps press down, straightening the arms until they are fully extended and at your side.
4. Descend back to the starting position on the floor, simply perform the movement in reverse. Perform consecutive repetitions on one side, then switch legs.

Start this one by performing the reps slowly, and master the form. Progress by performing more reps consecutively, and add a little speed. Don't cut range of motion short at either end. Make sure you finish the movement.

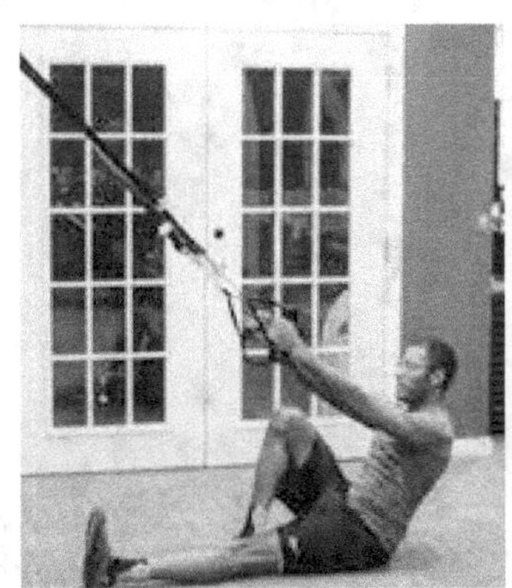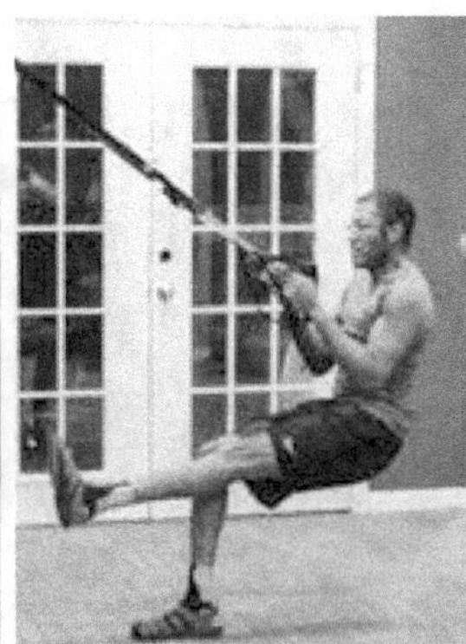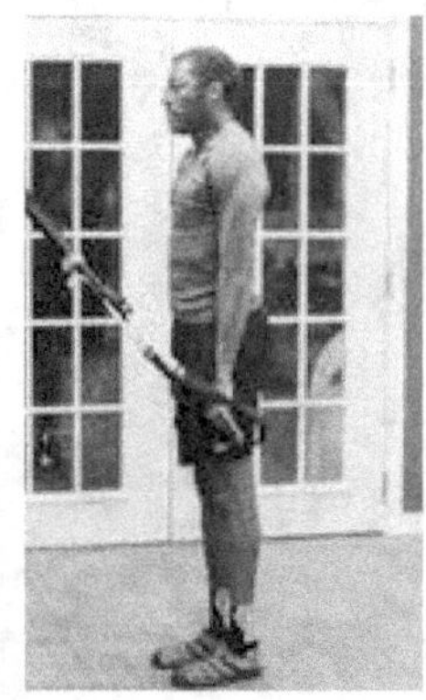

Bear Crawl   Whole Body

This is a great full-body and core movement. It will improve core as well as upper body strength, as well develop the motor pattern of arms and legs working together through a stable core.

Focus: Core and the front of the upper body.
No equipment needed

1. Start in a straight-arm plank position.
2. In one movement bring one arm forward in front of you, along with the opposite leg and foot.
3. Repeat the same thing on the other side, bringing your body forward over your hands and legs as you go.
4. Perform for a targeted amount of repetitions for each side, time, or distance.

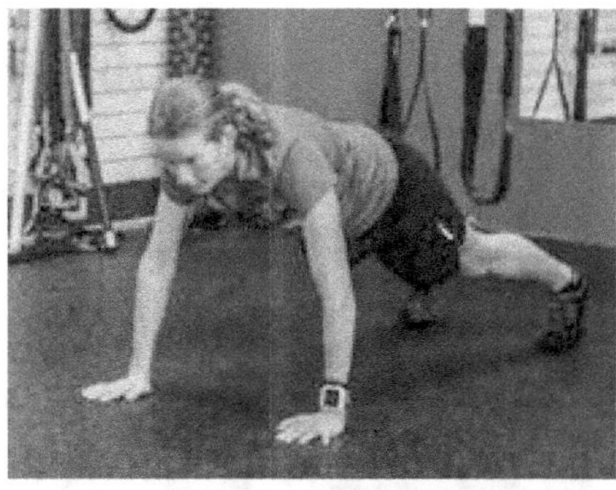

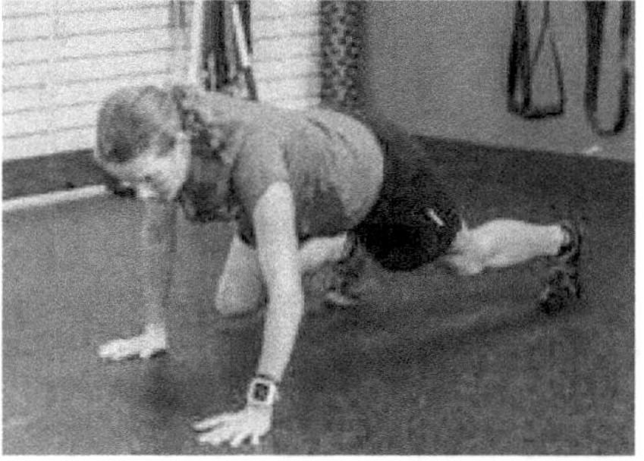

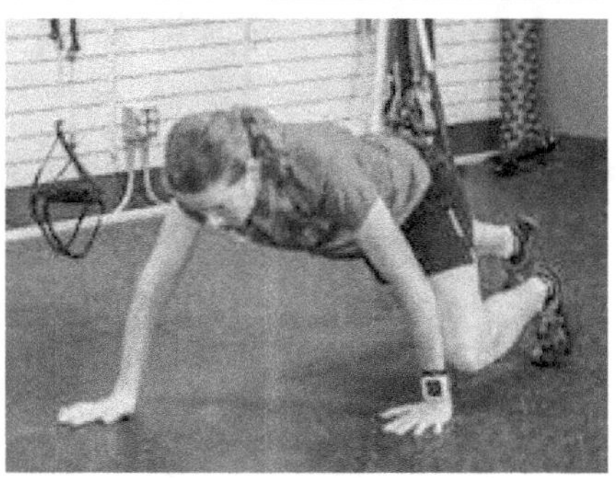

Keep a straight body, aiming to get your advancing knee close to the trailing arm each time. To increase the challenge, increase time or distance or reverse the movement and go backward.
Going forward and backward also works if you have a limited amount of space with which to work.

Suspended Burpee
Whole Body

This movement gives you a lot of bang for your buck. It's a challenging total-body movement that requires all-purpose strength, stability, and mobility.

Focus: Supporting leg and arms.
Setup: Straps fully extended and six inches off the ground.

1. Start by facing outward, standing on one leg with your other foot suspended in both cradles.
2. To start the movement, push the suspended leg back behind you as you lower your upper body to the ground
3. until your hands are on the ground in front of you. At this point, your supporting leg will still be underneath you with the knee bent.
4. Extend the bent leg behind you until that foot is next to the suspended foot. Your arms are now supporting your upper torso (as if you were going to do a push-up). Your body should be straight like a board.
5. To get back up, drive the unsuspended knee forward and back underneath you while keeping the suspended leg extended behind you. Now stand back up by returning your torso to upright as you push back through the front leg.

This exercise is about quality, not quantity. Use time or repetitions as a target goal for your sets, but don't get sloppy. If you feel you're losing your perfect form because of fatigue, stop.
Want even more? Add a push-up movement to the bottom of each repetition.

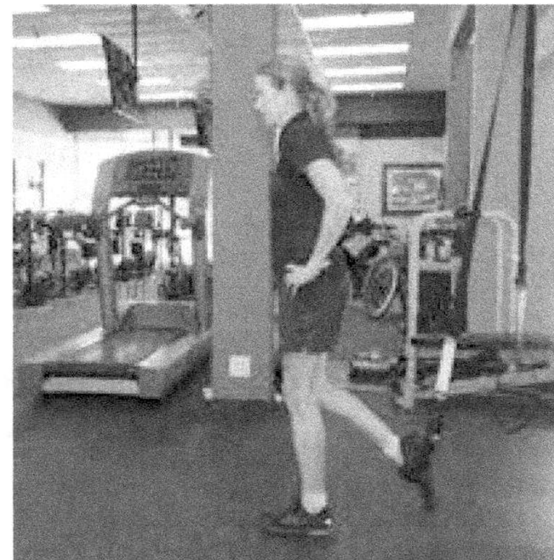

Suspended Burpee
(Continued)

Whole Body

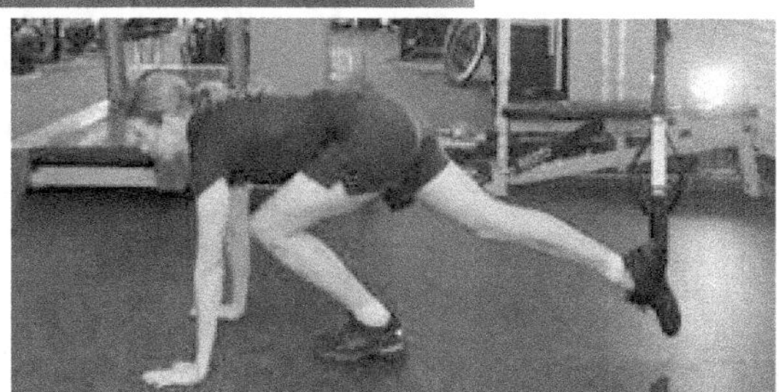

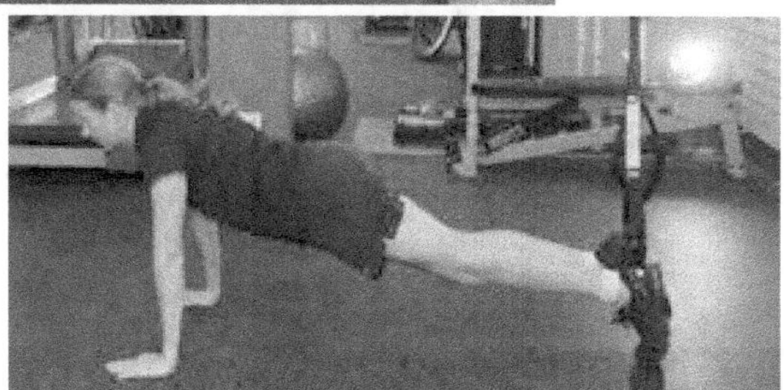

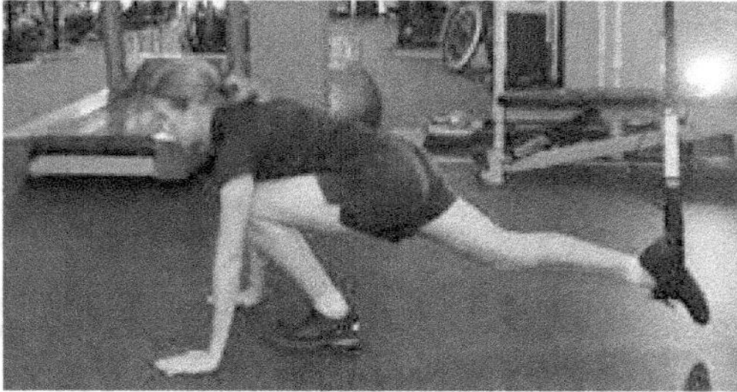

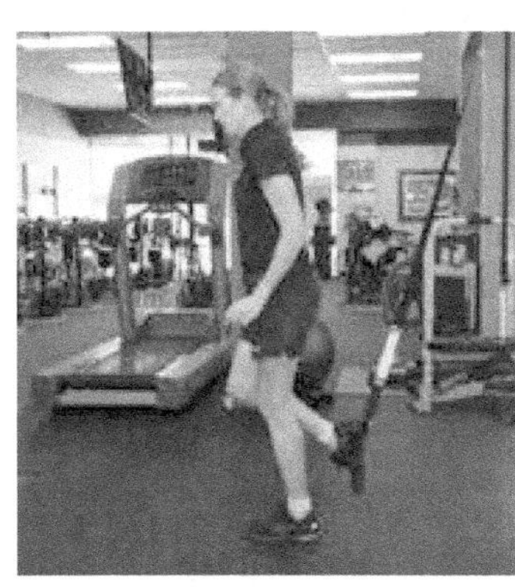

Full Get-Up Whole Body

This is a fundamental movement that requires maximum mobility, stability, and strength through the entire chain of the body. Make sure you have mastered the Half Get-Up before progressing to the Full Get-Up. Also, especially if you have never done this movement before, I suggest adding one progression step at a time.

Focus: Core and full body.

1. Lie on your back with one leg straight and the other bent. Point the arm on the bent-leg side straight up to the ceiling.
2. Start by lifting your shoulders off the ground as if you were doing a crunch, and continue ascending by pushing through the downed elbow. Keep your straight arm vertical and pointing at the ceiling the entire time!
3. When you get to the top of the half get-up, push through your arm and both legs to bring your hips off the ground and in line with the rest of your body
4. From this position, bring your extended leg back underneath you so you're now positioned on that knee. That knee should now be close to your grounded hand. Continue to keep your other hand pointed straight up.
5. Only at this point, allow your grounded hand to come off the ground as you bring your torso upright and vertical over your hips.
6. Push through the front leg to a standing position with your feet together.
7. Reverse the movement to come back down to the floor. Repeat all repetitions on one side, and then switch sides.

Whole Body

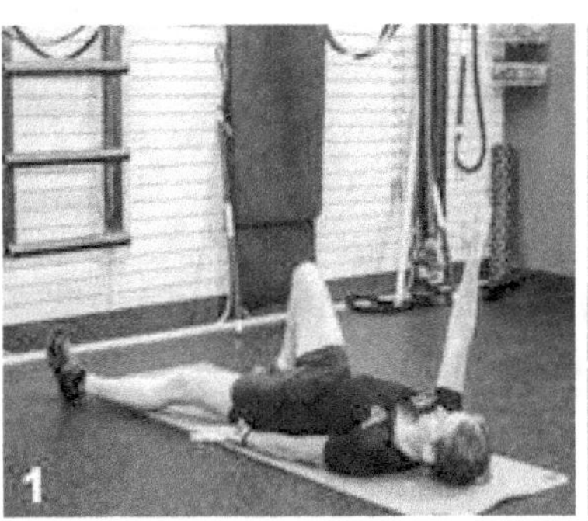 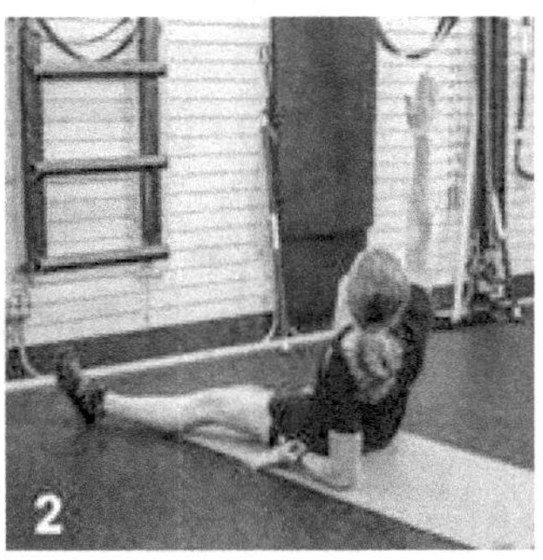

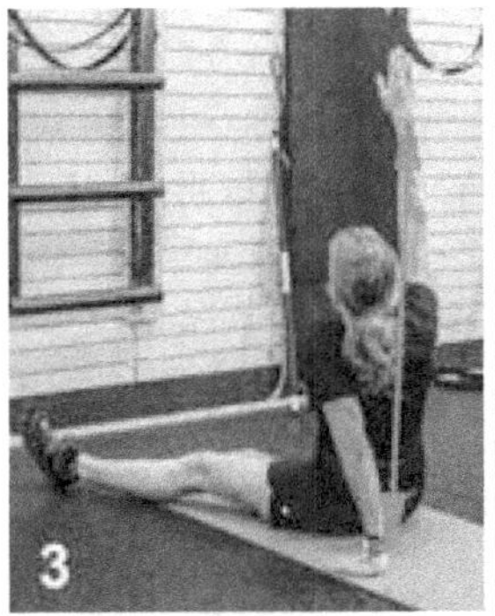 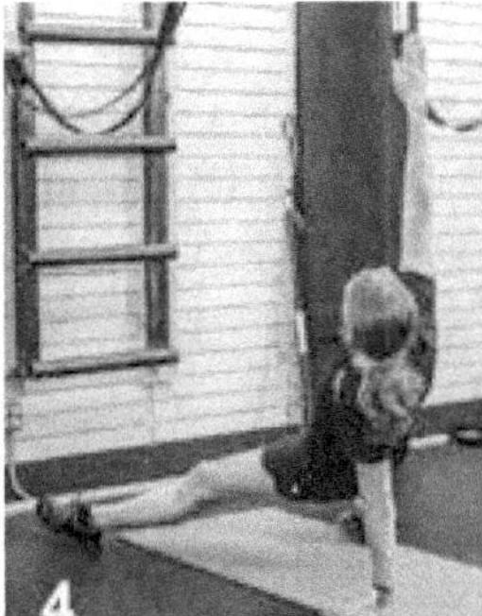 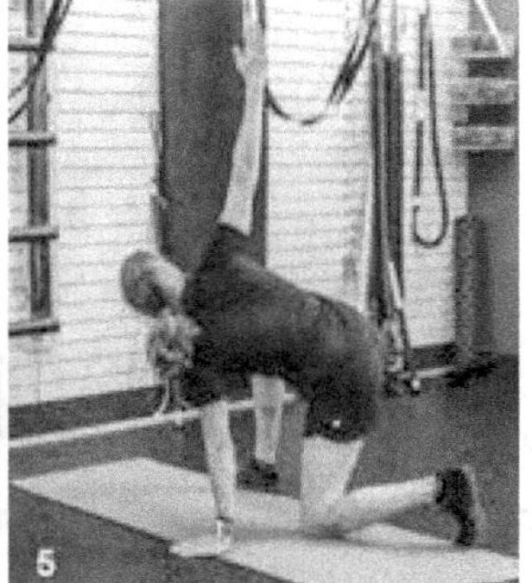

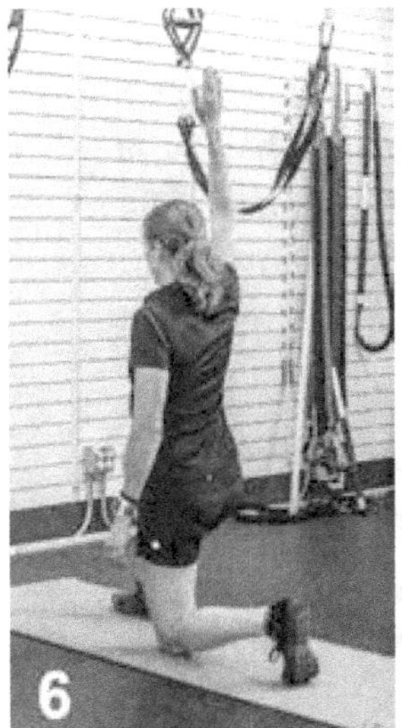 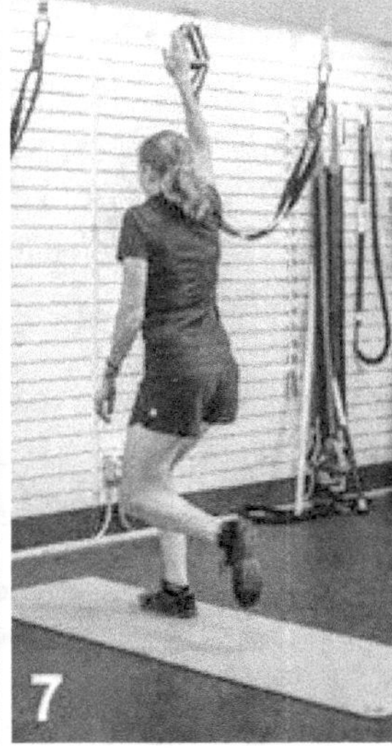 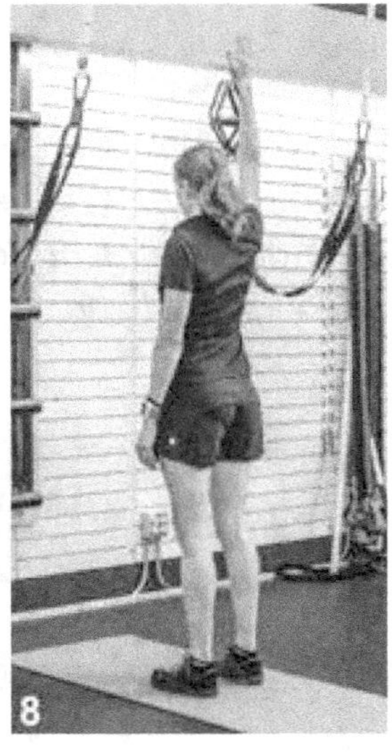

Spider-Man Push-Up Whole Body

This is a great upper-body and core movement that also requires hip mobility and strength. The simultaneous extension of one leg, and hip flexion of the opposing leg, develops strength and a movement pattern that is relevant to the pedal stroke. This movement will also help improve power transfer through the core, and hold a proper body position through fatigue and adverse elements.

Focus: Arms and core.
Setup: Straps fully extended and approximately six inches off the ground.

1. Start on your hands and knees facing away from the straps with the toes of one foot in both cradles. Your hands should be a little wider than shoulder width, at shoulder level.
2. Straighten both legs and push them back so you're supported by only your arms in front and the suspended leg. The free leg should still align with the suspended leg.
3. Go down into the push-up movement while at the same time pulling the knee of the free leg up toward your chest. Push back up as you extend the free leg back and move it back and in line with the suspended leg.

Keep your form! Don't sacrifice form for repetitions. Think quality over quantity. Keep the suspended leg actively extended to help maintain alignment. You'll feel the muscles in the front of the leg working hard to hold your position.

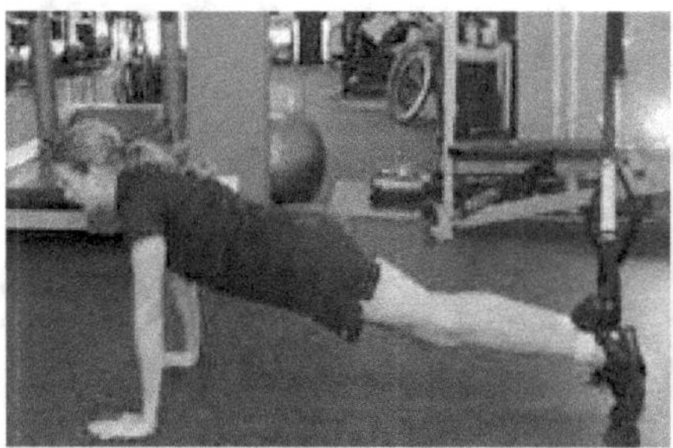
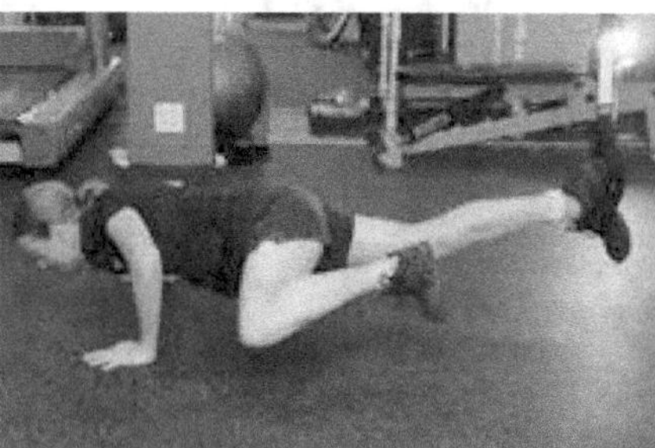

Chapter 10

Workout Programs

Foundational Level 1 Page 126
Foundational Level 2 Page 128

Run Specific Level 1 Page 132
Run Specific Level 2 Page 133

Foundation Workout Level 1

This program will help give you a solid foundation of general strength, stability, and better core engagement. Master this workout and you will become better conditioned to progress to more advanced and run specific suspension training workouts.

Frequency: Twice per week, in combination with additional endurance and flexibility training sessions.

Warm Up: Perform these at an easy to moderate intensity

Exercise	Targeted Area	Sets	Reps	Rest
Golf Rotation	Upper Torso	2-3	15 ea side	30 seconds
Squat Row	Legs and Torso	2-3	15	30 seconds

Summary of Program: Perform at a moderate intensity

Exercise	Targeted Area	Sets	Reps	Rest
Suspended Pushup	Chest/ Shoulders	2-3	15	30 seconds for all or as needed
Suspended Row	Back/ Biceps	2-3	15	
Split Squat	Legs/Hips	2-3	15	
Half Get Up	Core	2 ea side	10 ea side	
Front Squat	Legs/ Hips	2-3	15	

Golf Rotation

Keep one arm in place, and reach up and slightly behind you with the other arm, rotating your torso and looking in the same direction.

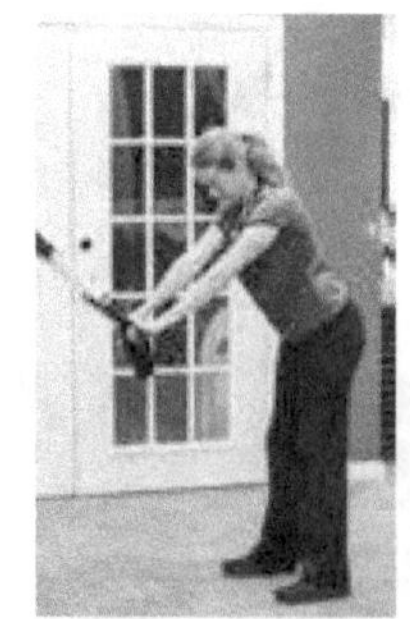
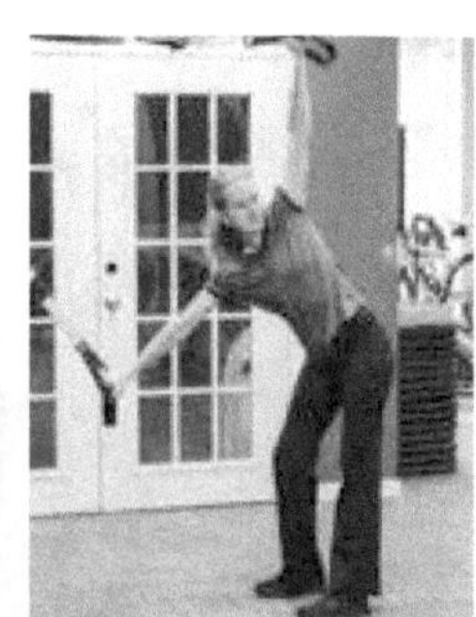

Squat Row

Lean back slightly on the straps. Sit down into the squat while extending your arms. Push yourself back up with your legs while also simultaneously pulling your upper body toward the straps.

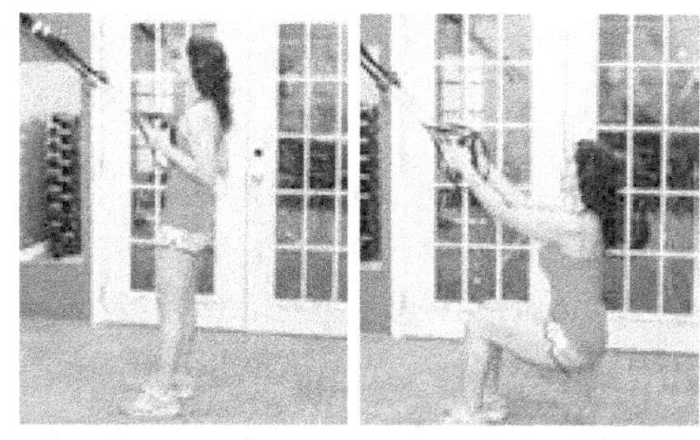

Suspended Push-Up

Keep a straight body position from your head to your feet. Lower your body until your elbows reach ninety degrees and are aligned with your shoulders.

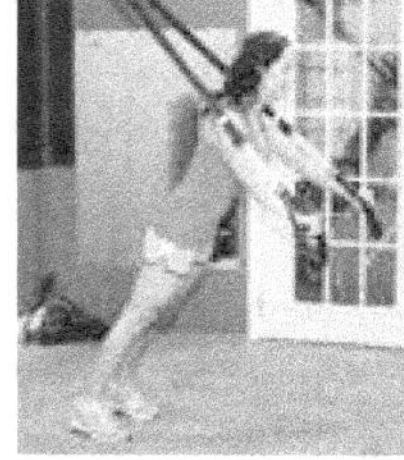
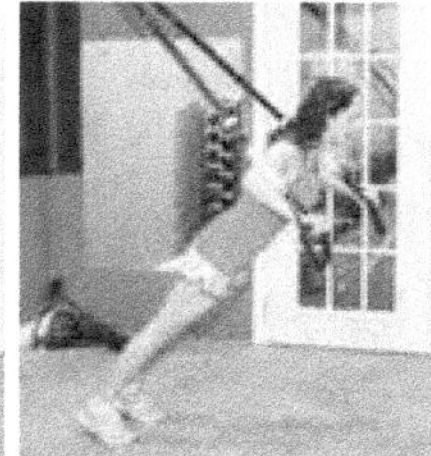

Row

Straighten your arms and lean back. Pull yourself up until your elbows are bent and at your side. Keep your body straight.

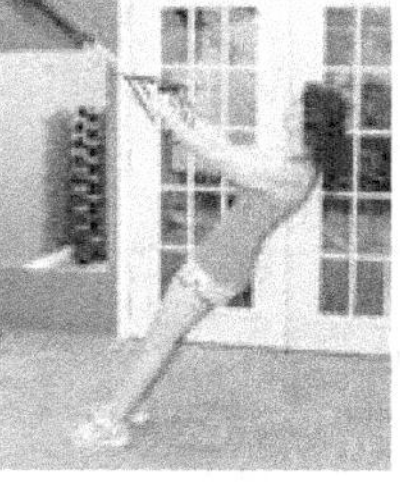
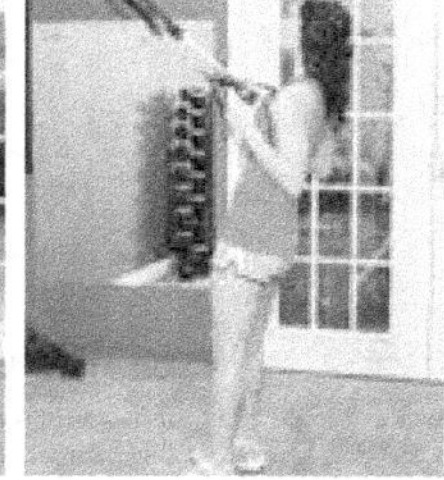

Split Squat

Take a large step behind you. Drop the back knee down toward the floor. Push back up through your back toe and the front foot.

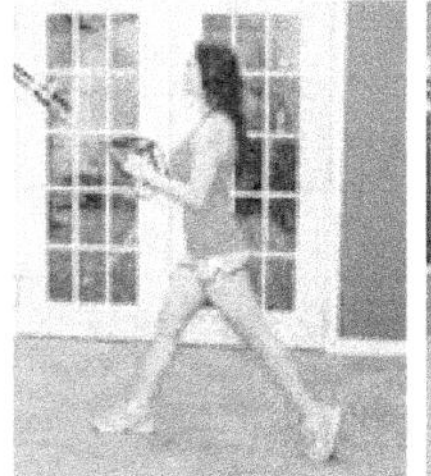
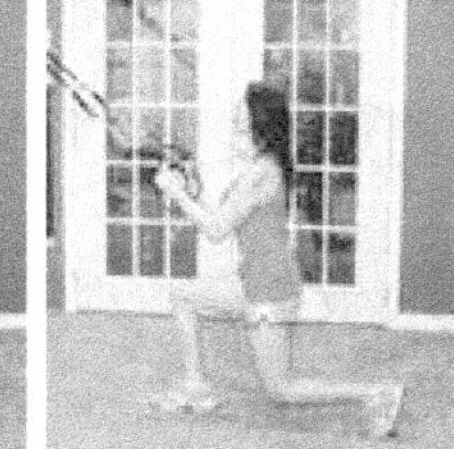

Front Squat

Lean into the straps with the handles in your armpits. Allow your knees to bend and your hips to descend back and down behind you toward the floor. Push back up from the bottom, continuing to lean into the straps.

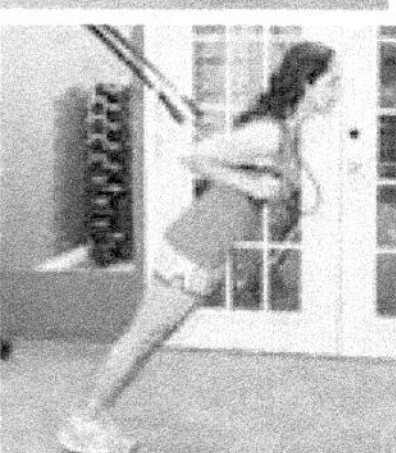
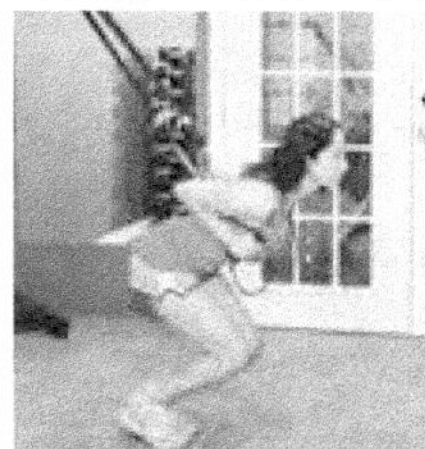

Plank

Raise your body up as one unit. Your body should form a straight line from shoulders to ankles.

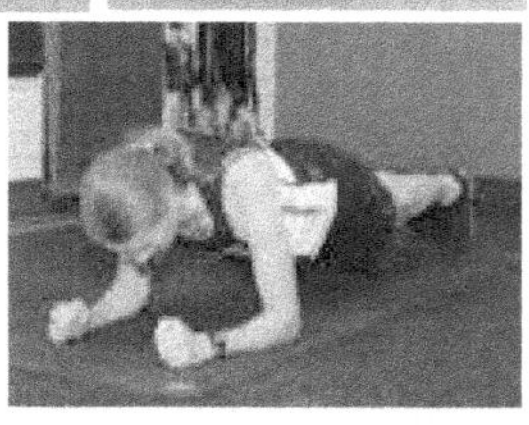

Foundation Workout Level 2

This program consists of more advanced movements than level 1, and movements that can also be progressed. The number of repetitions in some of the sets are lower because the resistance and difficulty of the movement is higher, which emphasizes strength development. If you're unable to perform one of the movements, step back to comparable movements in the level 1 workout ,and continue to work on progressing that movement at that level.

Frequency: Twice per week, in combination with additional endurance and flexibility sessions.

Warm Up: Perform at a moderate intensity

Exercise	Targeted Area	Sets	Reps	Rest
Squat Press	Full Body	2-3	15	30-60 Seconds
Suspended Get Up	Full Body	2-3	8 ea side	

Summary of Program: Perform at a moderate to hard intensity

Exercise	Target	Sets	Reps	Rest
Push Up - Feet Suspended	Chest and Shoulders	2-3	10-15	30 seconds for all or as needed
Suspended Pull Ups	Back and Biceps	2-3	10-15	
Side Plank	Core	2-3	15-30 seconds	
Sprinter Starts	Legs and Hips	2-3	10-15	
Reverse Flys	Upper Back	2-3	10-15	
Pike	Core	2-3	10-15	

Squat Press
Squat down with good form, as low as you are comfortable going. As you ascend, lean slightly into the straps and fully extend your arms above you. You may turn it into a squat press jump to increase the intensity

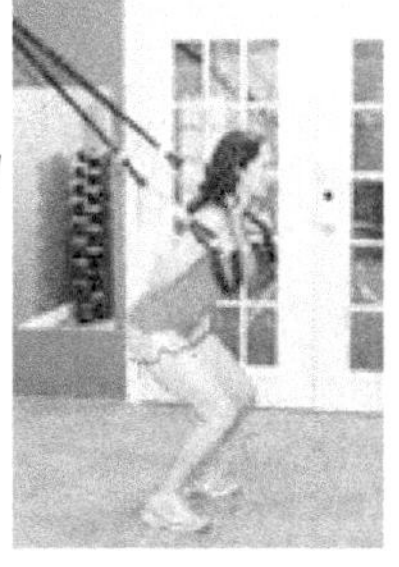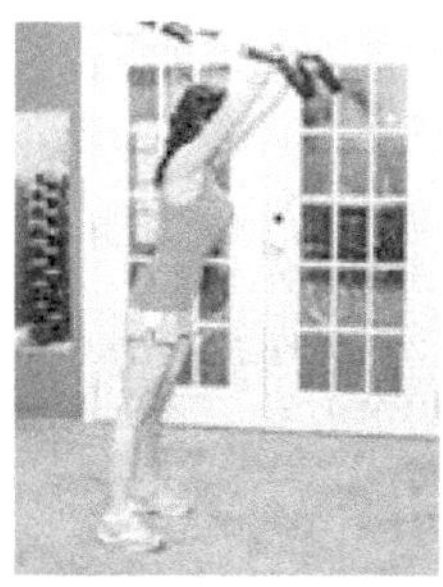

Suspended Get-Up
Start the movement by pushing through the hip of the bent leg, while simultaneously pulling yourself with your arms.
continue into a tricep press at the top. Descend by performing the movement in reverse.

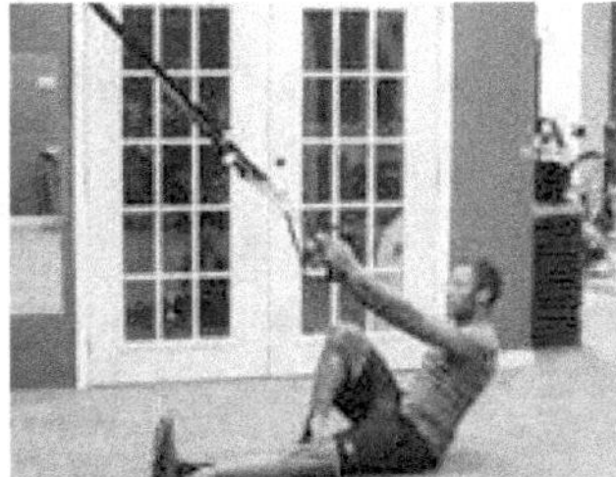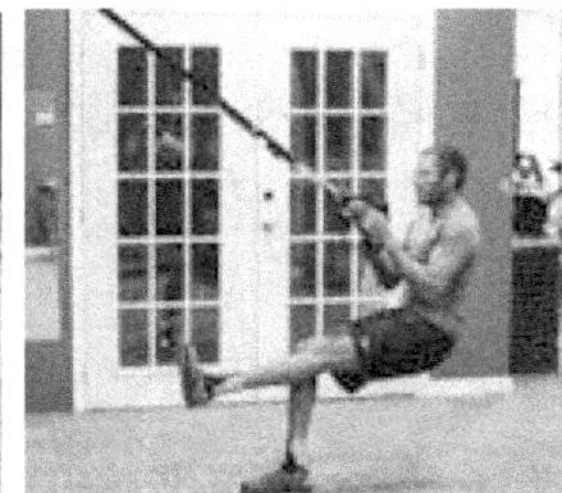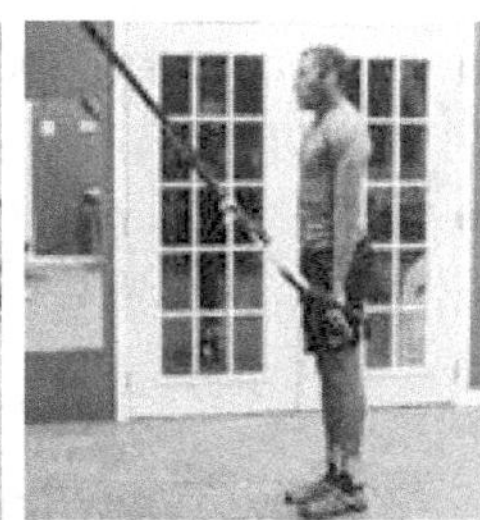

Push-Up (Feet Suspended)
At the bottom, push through the floor to raise your body back up to the starting position as one unit.

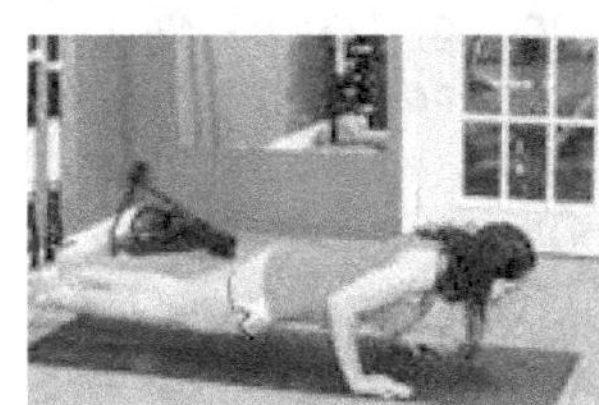

Suspended Pull-Up

Pull yourself straight up from the floor and until your chin is level with your hands. Think about pulling yourself over an imaginary bar.

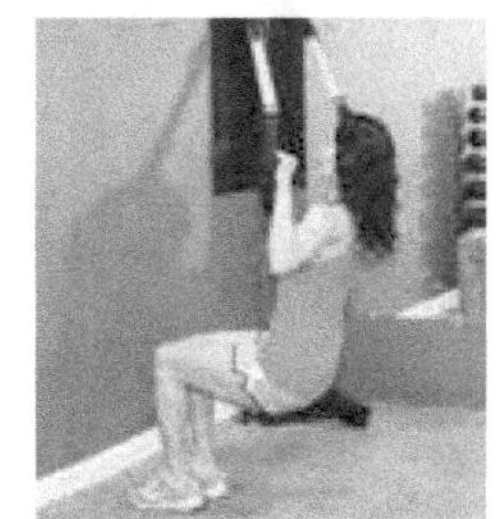

Suspended Side Plank
Your elbow should be directly underneath the shoulder, and the top leg should be forward. Lift your hips off the floor with your body weight supported by the arm and shoulder.

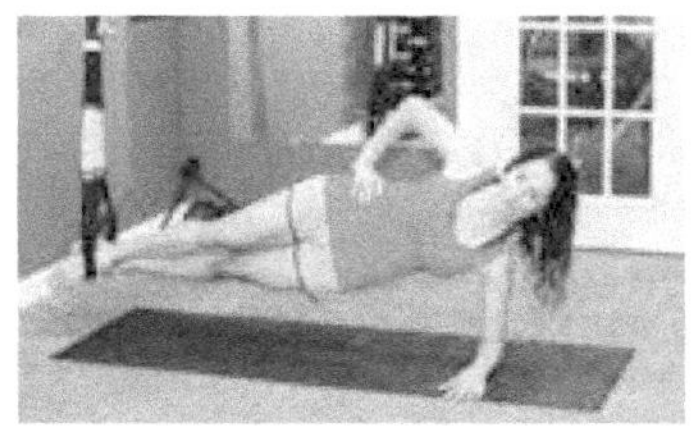

Sprinter Starts

Face away from the anchor with the straps underneath your arms, and lean forward into them. Take a large step back with one leg. Push back up through the front leg, and finish the movement by driving the knee of the back leg up and toward your chest. Alternate legs.

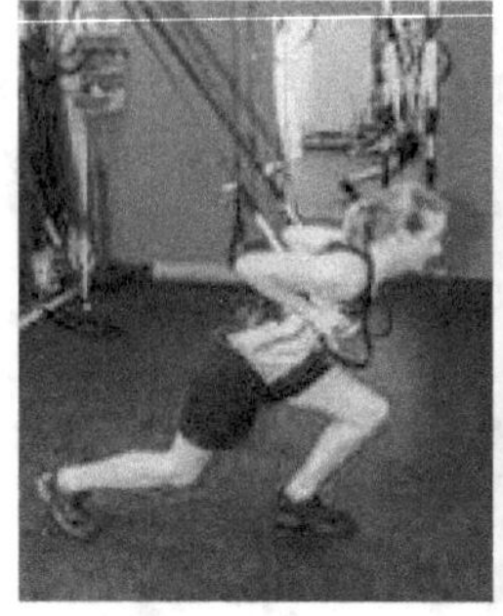
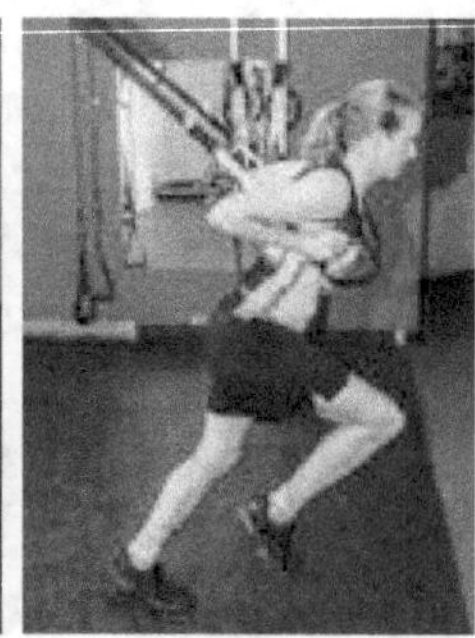

Reverse Fly

Face the anchor with your arms extended in front of you and a slight backward lean. Keeping the arms straight, open up the arms and bring them back to extend out from your shoulders. This will bring your body forward. Bring the arms back together to the front, maintaining arm extension and a straight body.

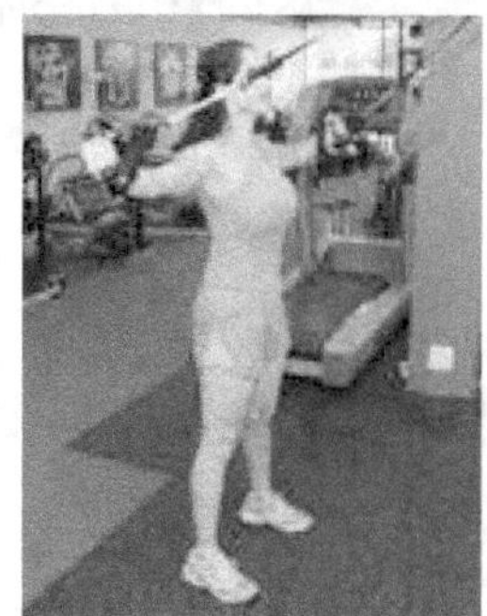

Pike

Face away from the suspended trainer on your hands and knees, with your toes in the cradles right underneath the anchor, and your hands underneath your shoulders. Straighten your legs and pull your legs toward your chest by driving your hips upward toward the ceiling.

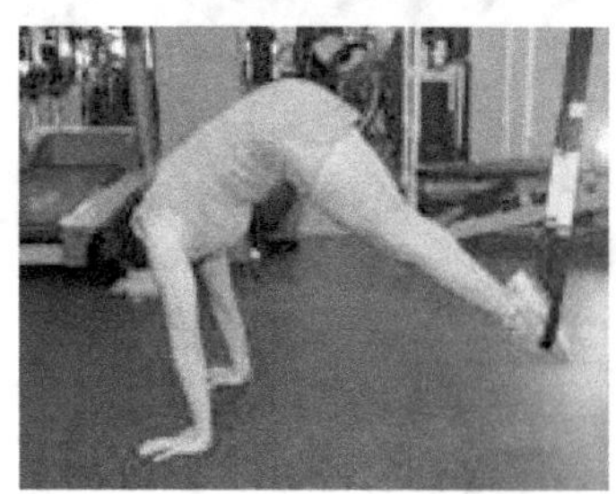

Cycling- Specific Strength Workouts

These circuits are short workouts that can be done alone, in combination with endurance workouts, or extended to longer workouts by adding more movements. Each circuit consists of a pushing, pulling, leg, and core movement. The level 1 circuit is appropriate for all levels. The level 2 circuit 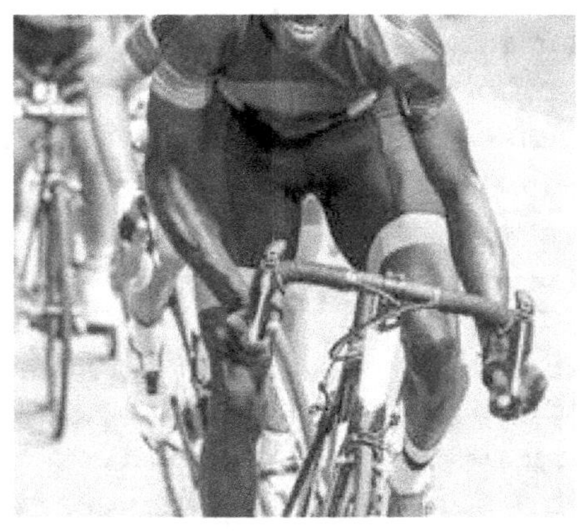 contains more advanced movements, and is for intermediate and advanced levels. If you're just starting a strength routine, you will benefit most by mastering the foundation workout first.

Although these workouts are cycling specific, they're not necessarily specific to where you are in your season, or your cycling discipline. Keep this in mind and adjust as needed to fit your program. See chapter 8 for more information on how to do this. These circuits are merely suggestions. Don't limit yourself to them or be afraid to substitute and progress movements. I chose to base the sets on time. Focus on intensity and quality of repetitions over how many you can get in during the time. You may also choose to base your sets on repetitions.

The workouts are designed to be shorter in duration as to complement your existing run training program. These may also be done on the same day as a cycling training session. Saying this, be sure to prioritize your sessions based on importance in terms of what you want to get out of them. For example, if a speed or anaerobic interval session is a key training session, you may want to perform the strength work either after the session or a different day. If you are working with a coach, I would also suggest consulting with them about how to best add the strength sessions to your existing individual training program.

Frequency: *Two times/week in combination with additional endurance and flexibility training sessions.*

Warm up *with fifteen minutes on a stationary bike or trainer if possible. Include three thirty-second spin-ups of high resistance and high cadence to get the oxygen levels higher in your muscles and your heart rate up.*

Level 1 Cycling Specific *Moderate to Hard Intensity Level*

Exercise	Targeted Area	Sets	Time	Rest
Suspended Push-Ups	Chest and Shoulders	2–3	30 seconds	30 seconds for all or as needed
Suspended Row	Back and Biceps	2–3	30 seconds	
Split Squat or Reverse Lunge	Legs and Hips	2–3	30 seconds	
Half Get-Ups	Core	2–3	30 seconds	
Plank	Core	2-3		

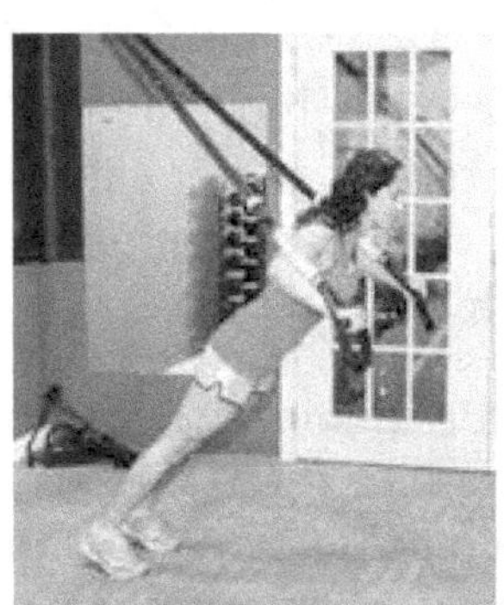
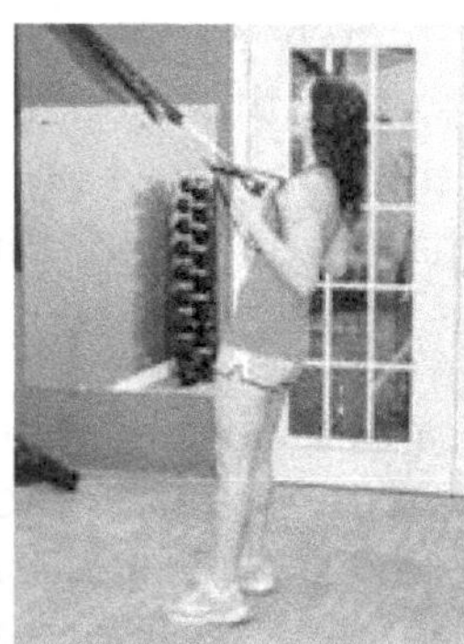
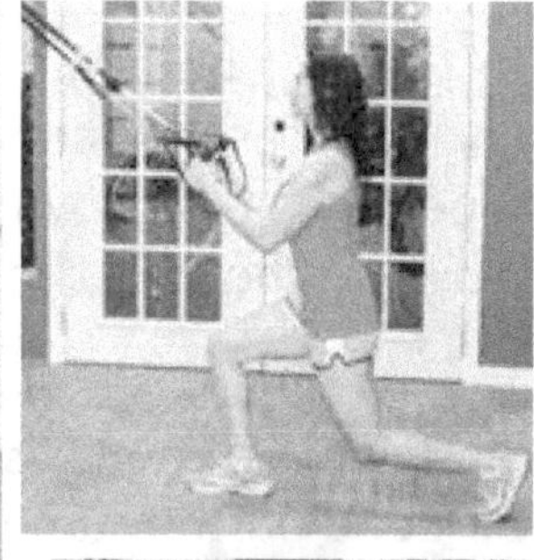
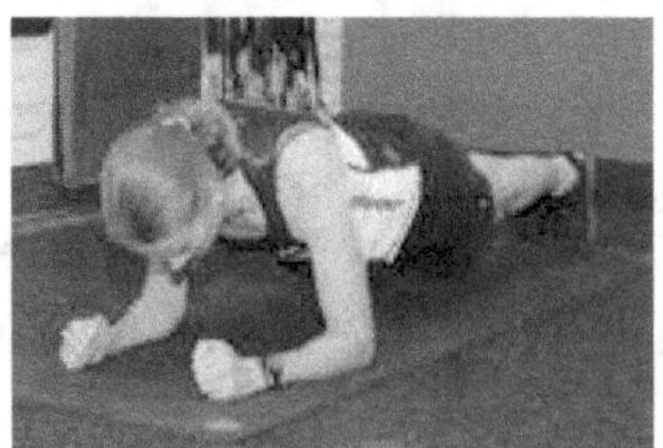
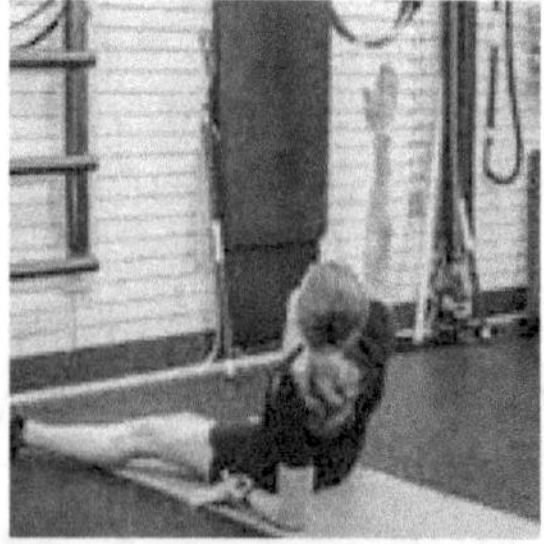

Frequency: *Two times/week in combination with additional endurance and flexibility training sessions.*

Warm up *with fifteen minutes on a stationary bike or trainer if possible. Include three thirty-second spin-ups of high resistance and high cadence to get the oxygen levels higher in your muscles and your heart rate up. .*

Level 2 Cycling Specific

Movement	Targeted Area	Sets	Time	Rest
Push Up- Feet Suspended	Chest and Shoulders	2-3	30 seconds	30 seconds or as needed
Suspended Pull-Ups	Back and Biceps	2-3	30 seconds	
Sprinter Starts*	Legs and Hips	2-3	30 seconds	
Atomic Crunch	Core	2-3	30 seconds	
Side Plank	Core	2-3	30 seconds	

**Side plank may be done grounded or suspended.*
***Sprinter Starts may be progressed to Sprinter Starts with Hop*

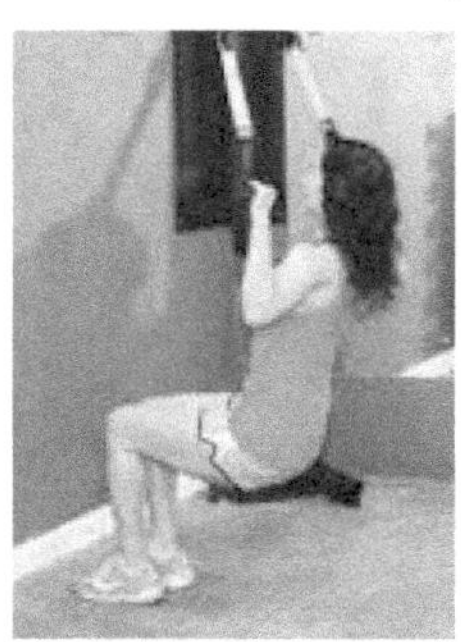
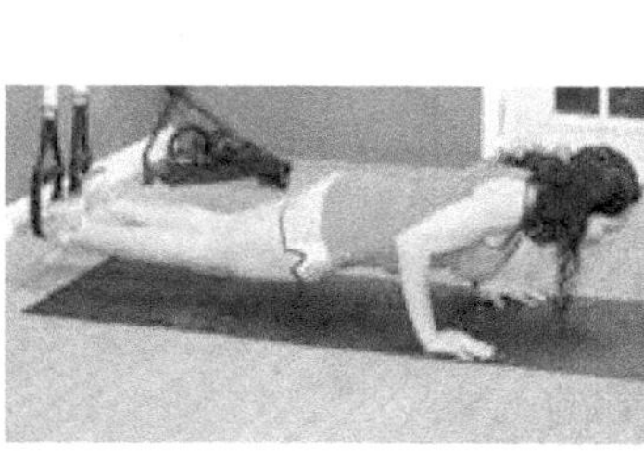
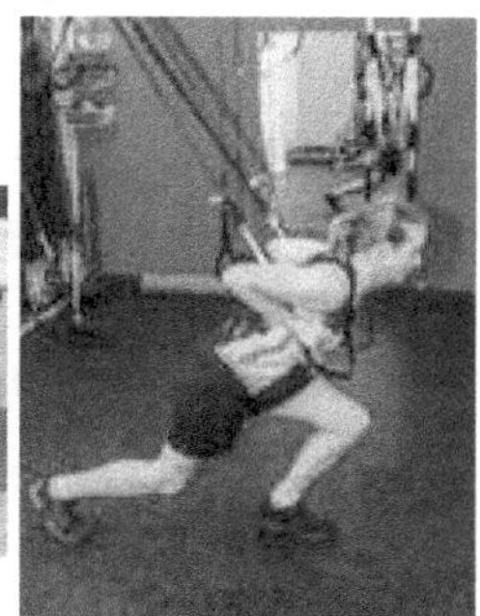
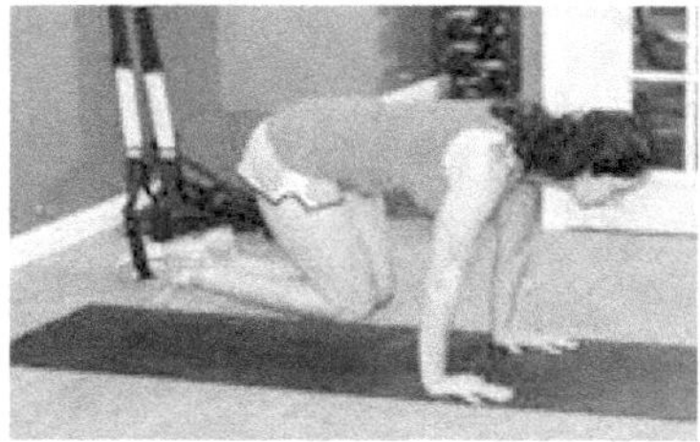
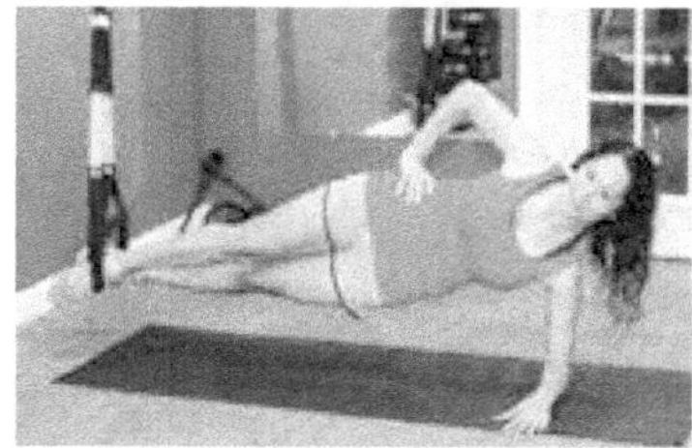

I hope you enjoyed this book and are feeling more confident and comfortable using your suspended trainer.

I also hope you are feeling the benefits of better strength and stability that leads to a strong, more fatique resistant run.

Feel free to contact me through the website below if you have any questions regarding this book or the information provided. You will also find additional resources located there for suspended training as well as other methods.

www.suspensionfitnessandbeyond.com

If you are ready to move forward in your fitness journey with suspension, please check out the ***Complete Suspension Fitness Book.*** There you will find and more information on additional aspects of improvement to your health. fitness, stamina and strength using a suspended trainer as your main tool!

References

Chapter 1

1. Byrne, Jeannette M., Bishop, Nicole S., Caines, Andrew M., Crane, Kalynn A., Feaver, Ashley M. Pearcey, and E. P. Gregory. "Effect of Using a Suspended Training System on Muscle Activation during the Performance of a Front Plank Exercise." *Journal of Strength and Conditioning Research* Vol. 28 (November 2014): 3049–3055.

2. Kibele, Armin, and David G. Behm. "Seven Weeks of Instability and Traditional Resistance Training Effects on Strength, Balance and Functional Performance." *Journal of Strength and Conditioning Research* Vol. 0 (October 2009) 1–8.

3. Snarr, Ronald L., and Michael R. Esco. "Electromyographical Comparison of Plank Variations Performed with and without Instability Devices." *Journal of Strength and Conditioning Research* Vol. 28 (November 2014) 3298–3305.

4. Gillette, Mike. *Rings of Power: The Secrets of Successful Suspended Training.* St Paul, MN: Dragon Door Publications, Inc., 2015.

Chapter 5

1. Yamamoto, Linda M., Jennifer F. Klau, Douglas J. Casa, William J. Kraemer, Lawrence E. Armstrong, and Carl M. Maresh. "The Effects of Resistance Training on Road Cycling Performance Among Highly Trained Cyclists: A Systematic Review." *Journal of Strength and Conditioning Research* Vol. 24 (February 2010): 560–566.

2. Paton, Carl D., and William G. Hopkins. "Combining Explosive and High Resistance Training Improves Performance in Competitive Cyclists." *Journal of Strength and Conditioning Research* Vol. 19 (April 2005): 826–830.

3. Jackson, Nathaniel P., Matthew S. Hickey, and Raoul F. Reiser. "High Resistance/Low Repetition vs. Low Resistance/High Repetition Training: Effects on Performance of Trained Cyclists." *Journal of Strength and Conditioning Research* Vol. 21 (January 2007): 289–295.

4. Bastiaans, J. J., A. B. van Diemen, T. Veneberg, and A. E. Jeukendrup. "The Effects of Replacing a Portion of Endurance Training by Explosive Strength Training on Performance in Trained Cyclists." *European Journal of Applied Physiology* Vol. 86 (November 2001): 79–84.

5. Bishop, D., D. G. Jenkins, L. T. Mackinnon, M. McEniery, and M. F. Carey. "The Effects of Strength Training on Endurance Performance and Muscle Characteristics." *Medicine & Science in Sports & Exercise* Vol. 31 (June 1999): 886–891.

6. Hickson, R. C., B. A. Dvorak, E. M. Gorostiaga, T. T. Kurowski, and C. Foster. "Potential for Strength and Endurance Training to Amplify Endurance Performance." *Journal of Applied Physiology* Vol. 65 (November 1988): 2285–2290.

7. Rønnestad, B. R., J. Hansen, I. Hollan, and S. Ellefsen. "Strength Training Improves Performance and Pedaling Characteristics in Elite Cyclists." *Scandinavian Journal of Medicine & Science in Sports* Vol. 25 (April 2015): e89–e98.

8. Segerström, Åsa B., Anna M. Holmbäck, Targ Elzyri, Karl-Fredrik Eriksson, Karin Ringsberg, Leif Groop, Ola Thorsson, and Per Wollmer. "Upper Body Muscle Strength and Endurance in Relation to Peak Exercise Capacity during Cycling in Healthy Sedentary Male Subjects." *Journal of Strength and Conditioning Research* Vol. 25 (May 2011): 1413–1417.

9. Maldonado, B. *Preferred Movement Patterns in Cycling*, Minneapolis: Langdon Street Press, 2010.

Chapter 6

1. National Institute of Arthritis and Musculoskeletal and Skin Diseases. "*Osteoporosis.*" http://www.niams.nih.gov/health_info/bone/osteoporosis/.

2. National Osteoporosis Foundation. "*Prevention: Who's at Risk?*" https://www.nof.org/prevention/general-facts/bone-basics/are-you-at-risk/.

3. Conroy, Brian P., and Roger W. Earle. *Essentials of Strength and Conditioning NSCA*. Champaign, IL: Human Kinetics. Chapter 4.

4. Brentano, Michel A., Eduardo L. Cadore, Eduardo M. Da Silva, Anelise B. Ambrosini, M. Coertjens, Rosemary Petkowicz, Itamara Viero, and Luiz F. M. Kruel. "Physiological Adaptations to Strength and Circuit Training in Postmenopausal Women with Bone Loss." *Journal of Strength and Conditioning Research* Vol. 22 (November 2008): 1816–1825.

5. Donald A. Chu. *Jumping into Plyometrics*. Champaign, IL: Human Kinetics, 1998.

6. Mosti, Mats P., Nils Kaehler, Astrid K. Stunes, Jan Hoff, and Unni Syversen. "Maximal Strength Training in Postmenopausal Women with Osteoporosis or Osteopenia." *Journal of Strength and Conditioning Research* Vol. 27 (October 2013): 2879–2886.

7. Almstedt, Hawley C., Jacqueline A. Canepa, David A. Ramirez, and Todd C. Shoepe. "Changes in Bone Mineral Density in Response to 24 Weeks of Resistance Training in College-Age Men and Women." *Journal of Strength and Conditioning Research* Vol. 25 (April 2011): 1098–1103.

8. Scofield, K. L., and S. Hecht. "Bone Health in Endurance Athletes: Runners, Cyclists, and Swimmers." *Current Sports Medicine Reports* Vol. 11 (November–December 2012): 328–334.

9. Lanye, Jennifer E., and Miriam E. Nelson. "The Effects of Progressive Resistance Training on Bone Density: A Review." *Medicine & Science in Sports & Exercise* Vol. 31 (January 1999): 25–30.

10. Nichols, Jeanne F., and Mitchell J. Rauh. "Longitudinal Changes in Bone Mineral Density in Male Master Cyclists and Nonathletes." *Journal of Strength and Conditioning Research* Vol. 25 (March 2011): 727–734.

11. Olmedillas Hugo, Alejandro González-Agüero Luis A. Moreno, José A. Casajus, and Germán Vicente-Rodríguez. "Cycling and Bone Health: A Systematic Review." *BMC Medicine* (December 2012).

Chapter 7

1. Fleck, Steven J. "Periodized Strength Training: A Critical Review." *Journal of Strength and Conditioning Research* Vol. 13 (January 1999) 82–89.

ABOUT THE AUTHOR

Tracy holds a B.S. in Biology and an M.S. in Human Performance from the University of Wisconsin at La Crosse, and is a certified strength and conditioning specialist (CSCS) through the NSCA. Tracy is a Level 2 USA Cycling coach and a Level 1 USA Triathlon coach. She holds a Level 2 Functional Movement Systems screening certification, which enables her to examine and assess basic movement patterns for dysfunction and make corrections. She also holds a TRX® Suspension Training Advanced Group certification.

In her spare time, Tracy's personal passion is training and competing in triathlons, road races, and criteriums. She has several age-group wins and podiums in triathlons, and podiums in the Texas Racing Cup series for cycling. She currently lives in Dallas with her husband, who runs Cycling Center Dallas, a wattage-based training facility for cyclists and triathletes. They share their house with many bikes, two crazy dogs, and one plant.

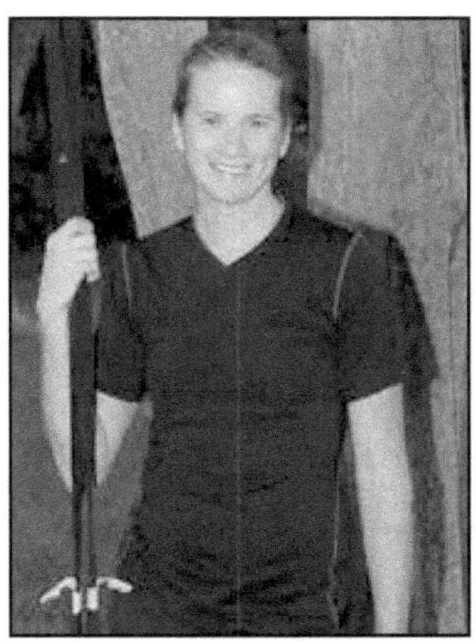

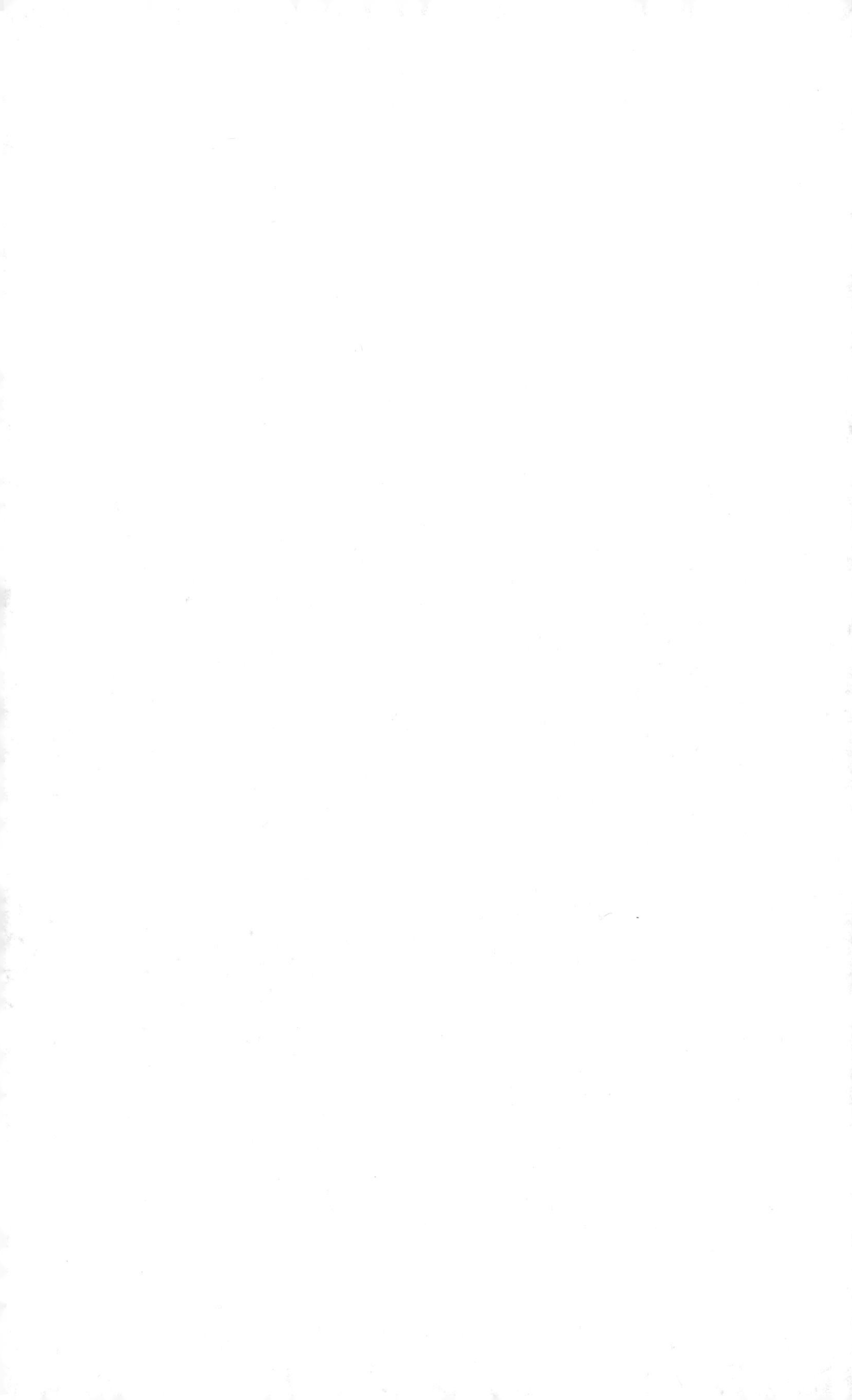